Provings of Vine

Vitis vinifera

A proving of two homeopathic remedies

White - Austria - Vitis vinifera folium
Peter König & Gerda Dauz, Eisenstadt / Vienna

Red - Germany - Vitis vinifera cum fructibus
1998 - 2003
Jürgen Weiland, Bonn

translated from German by:

Hilary Hampel, Merseyside, UK
Kurt Hampel, Mold, UK

Provings of Vine
Vitis vinifera – A proving of two homeopathic remedies

Peter König & Gerda Dauz
Jürgen Weiland

Translation:
Hilary Hampel, Merseyside, UK
Kurt Hampel, Mold, UK

Original English Edition.
Deutsche Originalausgabe by Fagus Verlag 2003.

Copyright © Fagus Verlag Jörg Wichmann, Rösrath 2004

1. Edition   June 2004
2. Edition   Dec. 2014
Printed by Books on Demand, Hamburg

FAGUS- Verlag, Jörg Wichmann
Eigen 81, D- 51503 Rösrath, Germany
e-mail: Jw@provings.info
www.provings.info

ISBN 3-933760-04-6

Table of contents:

'At the top of all remedies you find me, wine.
Wherever there is no wine, medicines are needed,
as all kinds of diseases appear.' [1]

Introduction: Why?

To conduct a homeopathic proving of wine, in order to create a specific remedy, has been an obligation, a temptation and a challenge for us for a number of reasons. Vitis vinifera is one of those 'minor' homeopathic remedies, which has been somewhat under-used in the shadow of much better-known remedies with a larger sphere of action. However, one could assume it would have a 'larger' sphere of action, not least because of it's cultural and historical significance as a noble companion throughout the evolution of human kind, in addition to symbol of peace and prosperity. The grapevine is also one of the prominent cultivated plants of both Burgenland and Rhineland, contributing to the shaping of their landscapes. It was in these habitats, in which the Vitis provings were analysed, evaluated and processed.

With the exception of one other homeopathic proving of an earlier date[2], we have, up to now (January 2003), no knowledge of any further medicinal trials based on Samuel Hahnemann's methods. To date there have never been any repertory rubrics listing Vitis, that were based on results from provings.

---

1 From a letter by the Apostle Paul to his student Timothy.
2 Karl-Josef Müller, Zweibrücken, published 1997, one of his 'under the pillow provings' with Vitis vinifera 200c (German Homeopathic Union), which refers however solely to dreams.

5

The grapevine and the juice extracted from its fruit have deep rooted associations with human beings and their cultures, very much like cereal crops. Wine was widely appreciated in ancient Egypt 5000 years ago and was attributed to the deities Isis and Osiris. Around 500 B.C. the Greeks are said to have introduced wine to Western Europe, and the Romans were responsible for it spreading throughout their empire. It's importance increased significantly since it became 'the blood of Christ' in altar wine.

There are some astonishing parallels between human beings and wine (and consequently the plant Vitis vinifera also), which became apparent only through our intensive studies: The plant requires similar climatic conditions to humans: they prosper like human beings in a warm/temperate climate - between 40 and 50 degrees latitude on our planet. Similar to human civilization, Vitis has spread (alongside people?) in the valleys of large rivers. Wherever there are grapevines, there are people and their culture. Under the right conditions, wine ages similarly to humans and also 'matures' with age. Both, vine and man need tender, loving care in order to develop, grow and mature. This care is particularly necessary with people who suffer from 'wine sickness' (alcoholism). – There are some striking linguistic links between man and wine (wine-language), which will be discussed in more detail later on in this book. And so, for our provers the proving facilitated in many respects an encounter with a familiar substance of familiar character, grown on native soil.[3]

Furthermore, it has been exciting and rewarding to discover aspects of the grapevine's 'psycho-activity'. In his book about psychoactive drugs, Rätsch includes Vitis as one of them. However, he did not support this with evidence. He holds 'alcohol' - as a secondary product at the end of the fermentation process - responsible for the widely known psychological effects, which are generally known, rather than the plant Vitis and it's constituents. It is important to be specific about the distinction between the homeopathic remedies Vitis, Alcoholus and Vinum. In this book we are also attempting to answer these complex questions from the perspective of homeopathic research, namely, as a result of our proving.

---

3 Here the question is whether one can expect differences in the type and intensity of a proving reaction, dependant upon the degree of familiarity with the proving substance. From the abundance of symptoms of a plant like Nux vomica we can rather conclude that the 'globalisation' of our Materia Medica occurred a long time before it became what we refer to it as today.

On August 31, 2002, the Austrian part of the Vitis vinifera proving had its world premiere at the 56th World Congress of the Liga Medicorum Homoeopathica Internationalis (LMHI) in Sibiu, Romania ('Vitis Vinifera – A new and surprising Remedy'). The first Vitis presentation in Austria took place on January 18, 2002 at the 'Vienna Homeopathy Lecture', which had been moved to Burgenland. On that occasion two of the female provers took part, as well as the manufacturer of the remedy and a vinologist; to all of whom we are very grateful.[4]

In this book we have incorporated two mutually inspiring Vitis provings as harmoniously as possible, one ('white wine') from Austria, the other ('red wine') from Germany. The sequence of the presentation is in accordance with the development of the plant Vitis vinifera itself (first the leaf, then the fruit), and the seasonal cycle (spring first, and then the autumn).

We have deliberately refrained from including a chapter on 'healing and consoling' through wine in the history of medicine (e.g. as in Plato and Hildegard von Bingen) to the present day ('prevention of heart attacks'). For one, there is sufficient literature on the subject available, but also specific 'Vitis effects' cannot be differentiated from general effects caused by alcohol (see below). Here the flavonoid preparations made from red vine leaves (Parthenocissus), which have a use in venous insufficiency as phytotherapeutic agents, are an exception[5] . We also felt it was not appropriate to explore Edward Bach's use of the grapevine as 'plant of the soul' (Vine and Grape) within the framework of this book.

---

4 Tapes of this lecture can be obtained through the authors or from Irl-Vertrieb (Peter Irl), 82131 Buchendorf, Neuriederstraße 8, Germany, or www.irl.de
5 We did not observe any noticeable venous symptoms in our proving.

The Plant Vitis Vinifera [P.K.]

Today it is generally acknowledged that neither the vine, nor the cultivation of wine originates in Greece, but in Asia Minor. I have already mentioned how it spread throughout Europe along the great river valleys in temperate grassland regions. There the vine can still be found occasionally in it's original 'wild' form as the woodland grapevine Vitis vinifera sylvestris.

Vitis vinifera is one of about 600 different varieties of vine plants (Vitaceae), which in turn belong to the dicotyledonous order of plants (Rhamnales). Therefore they are closely related botanically to the buckthorn family (Rhamnaceae). Cascara sagrada, Ceanothus as well as Rhamnus frangula (Alder Buckthorn), which are known in homeopathy and phytotherapy, also belong to this group of plants. Besides Vitis vinifera, the Boston ivy (Parthenocissus tricuspidata 'Veitchi', 'Wild Wine') is the best- known representative amongst the Vitaceae.

Vitis vinifera is a hardy woody perennial climbing shrub, which can grow for several hundred years. The vines have been said to grow up to 45 metres long (without human cultivating intervention), but they are usually 6 to 25 m in length. The bark typically peels off in strips. Vine roots go as far down as 20 metres, enabling them to collect water even during periods of drought. The tendrils are modified branches and are invariably positioned opposite a 3 to 5 lobed, dentated leaf. On every third node the tendril is conspicuously absent. The tendrils orientate themselves by touch (haptotropism). To a certain extent Vitis gains support by wrapping tendrils around parts of its own structure, wires and/or posts. This is accomplished by slowly rotating the shoots until they find something to grasp onto. The blossoms are rather inconspicuous, greenish-yellow in colour, exuding a pleasant smell during the flowering season (June, July). Wild-type vines are dioecious, have either male or female flowers, whereas cultivated Vitis vinifera varieties produce mostly hermaphroditic flowers. The multiple fruit, which develops from the flowers, is strictly speaking a panicle, but is generally known as 'bunch of grapes'.

Pests and pest control play a major part in the cultivation of wine. One of several known fungal diseases of the vine is the 'downy mildew' (Plasmopara viticola), which was brought across from North America, and is generally treated with sulphur. However, the vine's arch-enemy is phylloxera, widespread in these latitudes since 1870, especially root phylloxera. By grafting high quality shoots onto high quality mildew resistant American base-vines, the catastrophic problem could be kept under control. Unfortunately mildew seems to have made a recent recurrence in many places. The battles against flocks of birds raiding the vineyards, are fought by shooting salvos into the air and the use of low-flying aircraft, as happens in Burgenland prior to harvest time. This reminds us of war-like scenes used in pest control methodology.

Vitis vinifera is believed to contain high concentrations of copper, molybdenum, selenium and magnesium. I will not be exploring to what extent these elements also relate from a homeopathic viewpoint - i.e. whether Cuprum symptoms can be found in Vitis. However, I think it is worth mentioning here, so that readers can investigate this further.

Wine in Antiquity
- Mythology of Wine [J.W.]

*'Since the beginning of creation, wine has had the power
to illuminate the shadowy path that leads to the truth'* [6]

Wine in Antiquity

Alongside grains, wine is one of the earliest plants cultivated by man. More than 6000 years ago, nomadic tribes are believed to have fermented wild grapes to make wine. Together with olives and figs, grapes were among the first wild fruits to be domesticated. The earliest finds of tools and vessels allegedly used in winemaking date back to the 6th millennium B.C. They originate from the northern Caucasian regions and Persia of the 4th millennium. This is believed to be the birthplace of viticulture.

Wine first rose to prominence in ancient Egypt. During the rule of the Pharaohs, techniques of wine cultivation reached remarkable standards of perfection for the first time in history. The wine pressing methods of the ancient Egyptians survived for thousands of years.

---

6 Alighieri Dante (1265-1321), Italien writer and philosopher (The Banquet, The Divine Comedy)

The next step in the grapevine's conquest of the ancient world took place in ancient Greece. Wine became an important part of Greek culture during the 2nd half of the 2nd millennium B.C.

Wine was introduced into Southern Italy by Greek settlers. At the time, Pompeii was the centre of the wine trade. From there, wines were exported as far as Bordeaux. After the destruction of Pompeii, it was the Romans who brought about the dispersion of the grapevine throughout their empire.

Mythology

There is a close link between the history of wine and Dionysus, the Greek god of wine and vegetation. He was also the god of trees, often depicted as an upright wooden post wearing a mask. Green is the colour dedicated to him, symbolising nature's growth and vitality. Dionysus gave us wild, unfermented wine. It was used in religious ceremonies to bring about a oneness between mortals and the god they worshipped.

Dionysus is said to have been of Phrygian origin. In Phrygian, Dio means 'Zeus' and Nyos stands for 'young man'. He is also known as god of lust, love and ecstasy. He would frequently roam about with his entourage of nymphs, sirens and female worshippers of Bacchus. Dionysus symbolises everything connected with lust: lust for love, food & drink and dancing. He is the god who connects us with our instincts and animalistic nature. He is also considered the creator of theatre, the arena for rituals, where deep emotional and archetypal processes can be performed and processed.

Apollo, god of the sun, is the polar opposite of Dionysus. He is the god of day, creation, clarity and objectivity, the arts and sciences, as opposed to Dionysus, god of wine, dance and ecstasy. In Nietzsche's 'The Birth of Tragedy', we are to be convinced by Dionysian art of the eternal lust of existence. Should there be a development towards a predominance of Apollonian values - as was happening during Nietzsche's life in the 2nd half of the 19th century, which can, in his opinion, lead to a rigid, puritanical and corrupt state religion - then the vitality and cheerfulness of the child-god Dionysus, of springtime, can reawaken us to new life. In today's political climate, too, the Dionysian green movement, in tune with nature, is of great importance as an antithesis to the titanic (mechanised) forces.

We find quite varying representations and accounts of Dionysian mythology in classical literature. Some time after my Vitis study, I came across a story about Dionysus, which particularly reflects the above mentioned theme.

While on one of his numerous amorous adventures, Zeus, the greatest of the Olympian Gods, fathers a child with Semele, a mortal woman, who was the daughter of the king and queen of Thebes. Hera, Zeus's jealous wife, discovers the extramarital affair and seeks revenge. She entices Semele to ask her lover to reveal himself in all his divinity. Zeus, who had promised to fulfil each and every one of his lover's wishes, has no choice. He reveals himself in his full thunder-bolting glory, burning Semele to cinders instantaneously. At the time she is 7 months pregnant, and Zeus is able to save the child at the last moment. As a result of the lightning, the child has become immortal. Zeus sews the foetus into his thigh, and 3 months later his son Dionysus is born.

Since Hera's thirst for revenge is by no means quenched, Zeus chooses Hermes, the messenger of the gods, as an escort for the young god as a precautionary measure, and he is taken to the mythical island of Nyra. There he is brought up by local nymphs, disguised as a girl. Old Silenos, half man, half horse, who is often drunk, initiates him into the secrets of nature and of winemaking.

As a young man, Dionysus travels to Egypt, Asia Minor and India. He gathers together a great entourage of Satyrs, Silenes and Bacchantes. Wherever he goes, he instructs people in the art of winemaking, and women in particular devote themselves to Dionysian rituals, such as ecstatic dancing, music, alcohol consumption and sex.

However, many do not believe in his divine origins, and loathe his lustful Bacchanalia. For this rejection or contempt they were made to pay severely.

Thebes, Semele's city of birth, is ruled by King Pentheus, son of Agaue. Agaue is Semele's sister and doesn't believe her version of a divine conception. Instead, she has spread the rumour that Semele has become pregnant by a tramp, and her death was Zeus's revenge for using his name in vain.

King Pentheus wants to wash his hands of the effeminate, alleged god and his riotous cult. He throws Dionysus into prison. But Dionysus in turn destroys Pentheus' palace and forces him to attend the rituals. The king, disguised as a woman, makes his way to Mount Kithaeron, where preparations for the rituals are in full swing. Pentheus' mother Agaue is also there, amongst a group of women who are besides themselves in ecstasy. Whilst Pentheus watches the rituals, Dionysus causes people to focus their attention upon Pentheus. And this is how the god's bloody revenge is carried out: The women, in their divine drunkenness, believe the king to be a wild animal, and pull him to the ground. They tear him to pieces. Agaue impales her son's head on a pole and returns to the city triumphantly, where her father Cadmus brings her back to her senses. Only then does she realise what cruel fate she had been punished with by Dionysus. [7]

The experiences of provers 2 & 12 show how much the mythology of Dionysus is reflective of the Vitis study. In the same way as the Bacchantes tear Pentheus (representative of the anti-erotic warrior class) to pieces and Agaue impales his head, our female provers dreamt about cutting off heads or faces (as can be seen in the proving journals). It is interesting that through the effect of the proving remedy these female provers opened up and became more communicative and cheerful.

Face - Mask - Persona - Shadow
In vino veritas

On a variety of illustrations Dionysus is depicted with a 'mask' held up high (see cover).

A strong resonance with this theme was demonstrated in two female provers' dreams. In a sense, by cutting off the faces, people's masks fall off. It is interesting that after the 'masks' came down the two provers experienced an opening up in themselves psychologically. They stuck with what felt right for them to a greater extent, and as a result of that discovered their true face.

In psychoanalysis, the persona plays a considerable part in the inner psychological functions of revealing and concealing the self: Our adaptation to society is achieved by developing part of our personality, which C. G. Jung called 'persona'. This 'persona' was known as the mask worn by actors in classical antiquity.

---

7 Ton van der Kroon: Die Rückkehr des Löwen (The Return of the Lion)

'The persona is therefore a functional complex which came about for the sake of conformity or convenience, but is not the same as one's individuality'.[8] Hence the mask also has to do with conforming to parents and society in general: behaving as is expected. If the persona is attached too firmly, then the individual's life becomes very narrow and rigid (Apollonian-Dionysian conflict). When the mask drops, we can see the less attractive, often suppressed characteristics, which we like to banish into the shadows. However, when these aspects are integrated and given full expression, then our life can become brighter and more relaxed - as was the case for our Vitis provers. Dealing with our persona in more creative ways is, in my view, one of the main areas of application of Dionysian mythology and the deeper healing powers of Vitis vinifera.

Death and Resurrection

In various mythological representations Dionysus often embodies the cycle of death and resurrection. On one occasion, Hera revengefully ordered the Titans to abduct and kill young Dionysus. His limbs were torn apart, and he was then roasted and eaten. However, Athena found his heart and Zeus managed to restore his limbs.

Dionysus, like the vine, supposedly died each year, and was resurrected only after the first shoots appeared in spring. [9]

His cult is one of the many forerunners of a resurrected deity, from which Christianity developed later (Altar wine - Eucharistic celebration).

---

8 Carl Gustav Jung: the Collected Works of CG Jung, volume 6

9 Morgan J. Roberts: Myths and Legends of Ancient Greece and Rome

Vitis vinifera proving

(Folium vitis viniferae - White wine from Burgenland, Austria) [P.K. & G.D.]

Proving procedure & general conditions

The provers were previously students on a homeopathy course at the University of Vienna who had volunteered to take part in the proving (P.K., October 1990 - June 2001). Following a written pre-anamnesis, by means of a questionnaire devised by Hans Jörg Hee, St. Gallen, we eventually chose 15 provers, aged between 23 and 57: students, doctors, lay persons. They consisted of 9 female, 6 male (see Table 1).

During the proving, each prover was allocated a consecutive number followed by the code 'm' or 'f', depending on whether they were for male or female - in order to assist us in assigning particular proving symptoms to individual provers within the context of this book.

The remedy was chosen at random from a list of 8 pre-selected remedies that would be interesting to prove. Pharmacist Robert Müntz, Remedia (Eisenstadt) potentised it from the 3c trituration in Hahnemannian fashion, up to 30c. In our proving this was the 3c trituration of leaves from a 12 year old Vitis white wine plant, at first identified as a Grüner Veltliner, from the producer's vineyard, which had been grafted onto a base vine. Unfortunately we encountered unforeseen difficulties during our attempt to make an exact botanical vinological classification. According to later findings, we can assume the leaves to have been those of the 'White Burgundy' variety.

In March 2001, following the written pre-anamnesis by means of the above mentioned questionnaire, the provers received the remedy in a 30c, together with instructions to take it daily, until symptoms appeared, then stop, and perhaps repeat the process once more. The period of administration varied from 4 to 20 days. We consciously abstained from using placebo phases at any stage during the proving. Records of the provings were kept during administration and for at least 3 weeks post-observation. Personal post-anamnesis observations were collected afterwards.

Right until the end of the analysis and evaluation (incl. post-anamnesis) the proving was conducted double-blind, i.e. neither we as the evaluators, nor the provers, knew the identity of the proving substance. However, at the end of our editing of the proving we were able to identify Vitis amongst a list of 8 pre-chosen remedies as the most likely one, as a result of the actual symptoms.[10]

The evaluation itself was carried out according to a point-scheme which had previously been used successfully during homeopathic provings. Between 0 and 3 points are awarded in each of 5 categories for reactions and symptoms: Mind, Body, Generalities, Dreams and Curative response. The maximum being 15 points. From our 15 provers we rated 7 (amongst them just 1 male!) as having been sensitive to the remedy, with between 8 - 10 points each. From previous experiences, when extracting fundamental insights into proving remedies we know that those provers who respond the strongest (highlighted in grey in Table 1) are capable of giving an accurate account of the qualitatively most important symptoms and indications. This does, however, by no means imply that the individual symptoms of the other provers deserve no attention. The number in the 3rd column denotes the provers' self-evaluation according to the intensity of their reaction to the proving substance.

---

10 Owing to the lack of familiar Vitis symptoms this was however only possible via the signature-like content of our prover's dreams - see further on in the book.

Proving III/ 2001								
prover	time	responder 0-3 pt	reaction 0 - 3 pt.					sum of pt.
			mind	body	gen.	dreams	healed	
1 W	4	3	~	3	2	3	~	8
2 W	20	2	~	~	2	~	~	2
3 M	9+1	?	~	?	~	~	~	~
4 W	7	3	2	2	3	2	~	9
5 M	11	?	~	~	?	?	~	~
6 M	10	2	~	~	2	2	~	4
7 M	10	1	1	~	~	~	~	1
8 W	4	3	2	2	2	2	1	9
9 W	8	2	~	2	~	1	~	3
10 W	5	3	2	3	3	~	2	10
11 W	10	3	3	1	3	~	3	10
12 M	3+7	1	[1]	1	[1]	~	~	1+[2]
13 M	6	3	3	3	1	~	1	8
14 W	5+1	2	~	2	1	2	~	5
15 W	20	3	2	2	3	1	1	8

Vitis vinifera

Table 1

All of the provers' *first-hand accounts* of Vitis are shown in *italics* in this work.

Prover 13m, 24 years old, medical student
Flatulence, but a 'pleasant experience'.

As thematic introduction into the results of our proving we would like to quote prover 13m's impressive account in it's entirety followed by a short commentary, having taken 6 doses of Vitis 30c.

16.3. Remedy administered 8.00 am.
17.3. Remedy administered 9.00 am.
18.3. Remedy administered 7.00 pm.
Considerable flatus, loud and extremely foul-smelling, started in afternoon, worse in the evening.
19.3. Remedy administered 8.00 am.
Flatus absent in the morning, recurring again in the afternoon, worse in the evening.
Verbal attack from a woman in the underground (around 10.00am), but I didn't turn away, as I usually would have done. Instead I snarled back at her quite brusquely. Was very surprised about it myself, was this a reaction to unfair criticism?
20.3. Remedy administered 11.00 am.
Flatus as above,< after eating, in the evening> in the morning.
Dull pain in left forearm, radiating, sudden onset and decline. The pain then moved quickly to the right occiput and then disappeared (around 4.30 pm). Pressure and warmth have no effect.
21.3. Remedy administered 8.30am.
Flatus continues.
A similar situation as in the underground where I was at the till in the restaurant in the General Infirmary and where I felt I had been treated unfairly. Instead of suppressing my frustration or anger, suddenly, without thinking, I vented them. (13m/6)
Pain in various parts of the body, comes and goes very quickly, ie headache left temple for approximately _ seconds , like a prick or electric current.
22.3. No remedy administered from this point.
23.3. Flatus has subsided.
24.3. Heartburn after eating chilli (never have otherwise) from 9.00 pm until 11.00 am the following day, constant feeling as if something is pressing on my breastbone, really strong sensation of burning in the back of the throat above the larynx. Feels like my stomach has ceased up.
3.4. After an afternoon snooze wake around 3.00 pm and feel totally disorientated. Can't see what time it is on the clock. Keep thinking it's 9.00 in the morning and that I should have been at work an hour ago, then start to panic because I've been irresponsible. This lasts for about 2 minutes and only then do I realise that I have only been asleep for about half an hour and that everything is ok.
5.4. Identical situation as on 3.4; even occurs at the same time.
Overall, during this time, I have felt well in myself, full of energy, very self confident, was in a good frame of mind, and I managed to get a lot done. Thanks for the pleasant experience.

Our 24 year old prover is a blonde, pale-skinned, cautious young man, who doubts his own abilities; has anticipatory anxiety, and suffers a lot with erythrophobia (and, incidentally, prefers beer to wine), had a special encounter with Vitis, which he found pleasant.

It enabled him to have 'a very productive time' (original text from the proving notes) and opened up new areas for him. He experienced the release of a kind of impulsivity ('Acting without having to think about it for long'), which was new for him, particularly when he felt he had been treated unfairly. Some time after the proving was over this behaviour returned to 'normal' again. The combination of 'suppressed anger' and flatulence ('letting off steam!') would certainly have any homeopath thinking of Lycopodium. Regarding the flatulence, that became prominent in the proving, he comments that he had never noticed this before and he stopped taking the remedy because of this symptom. He couldn't put this down to being a result of external circumstances e.g. dietary influences. A side note: Calcium lacticum was the remedy that I (P.K.) prescribed for him as a constitutional remedy one year after the proving, when he presented with pharyngitis, with extreme swelling in the lymph nodes in the neck, which manifested at the time of his forthcoming new job. He responded very well to the remedy.

Selection of symptoms from the proving

The responses of those provers who were sensitive to Vitis vinifera were deep, far-reaching, and to some extent caused strong and reproducible changes - both psychological and physical. Whereas there are several demonstrations of gratitude for the positive proving experience (curative response, improvement in energy, more able to cope with life situations, ...), there was only one negative experience (prover 10f - toothache, sleep disturbance, which was also transmitted to her breast-fed baby, resulting in family conflict!) which required treatment and the antidoting of her proving symptoms (with Sepia). We have quoted Prover 1f's account as it illustrates other similar reports from the proving.

'I was quite surprised that I actually developed symptoms this time, as nothing happened during the first two provings I participated in. I was very happy to know that the pillules definitely weren't placebos'.

We have attempted to arrange this chapter in as practical a manner as possible. Individual quotes from the proving records have been classified according to a particular theme (heading) and (prover) number. At the end of each symptom we have included the prover's number. The number following the forward slash refers to how many days after taking the first dose of the remedy the symptoms occurred. 'P' means post-proving phase, e.g. 22P means the 22nd day from the beginning of the proving, from the time the first dose was administered, whereby in this case the observation of the symptom fell in the period following the last dose of the remedy. An ' F' means that the respective observation is a result of a follow-up consultation, which often occurred up to a few weeks after the last dose of the remedy. We decided not to separate curative symptoms from the rest. Underlining in the dreams stems from the provers, as also any other emphasis. ('C') refers to our comments on individual symptoms. The striking change in provers' energy has been given a chapter of it's own, following on from the general symptoms.

Mind

Calm, composed , peaceful [11]

Noticeable calmness and composure. (15f/ 2)
Extremely calm. (15f/ 3)
Noticeably calm and composed. (15f/ 5)
Extremely calm, well-balanced and composed. (15f/ 7)
Dream: large frogs that were croaking away happily. All in all, a very peaceful feeling. (5m/ 6)

Bad tempered, quarrelsome, annoyed [12]

Grumpy, everybody and everything is getting on my nerves. (8f/ 3)
In a bad mood all of a sudden, incredibly irritated by minor things. (8f/ 4)
Notice that I am sometimes being very unfair, but can't stop myself from being cross (start a quarrel suddenly, am really quarrelsome).13 (8f/ 4)

Sudden anger

In a bad mood all of a sudden. (8f/ 4)
Impatient, sudden annoyance building up, very easily offended and hurt (could have cried over the most trivial things). (10f/ 4)
I was under verbal attack from a woman in the underground (around 10.00am), but I didn't turn away, as I usually would have done. Instead I snarled back at her quite brusquely. Was very surprised about it myself, was this a reaction to unfair criticism? (13m/ 4)
A similar situation as in the underground, where I was at the till in the restaurant in the General Infirmary and where I felt I had been treated unfairly. Instead of suppressing my frustration or anger, suddenly, without thinking, I vented them. (13m/ 6)

---

11 The 'harmonious atmosphere' and serenity in the aforementioned Vitis proving by Karl-Josef Müller were also important symptoms.

12 Karl-Josef Müller: Irritability, observed in several provers.

13 Farokh Master, Bombay lists Vitis under 'Dictatorial, domineering' and 'Censorious, critical' (F. Schroyens: Synthesis). In a written reply to the author (P.K.), dated 10.12.2002, he mentions doing so as a result of clinical observations (with a patient he had prescribed Lycopodium for beforehand). Studying the Bach flower remedies also helped him in his understanding of Vitis.

Easily insulted, hurt

Impatient, sudden annoyance building up, very easily offended and hurt (could have cried over the most trivial things). (10f/4)

More assertive

Verbal attack from a woman in the underground (around 10.00am), but I didn't turn away, as I usually would have done. Instead I snarled back at her quite brusquely. Was very surprised about it myself, was this a reaction to unfair criticism? (13m/4)

A similar situation as in the underground where I was at the till in the restaurant in the General Infirmary and where I felt I had been treated unfairly. Instead of suppressing my frustration or anger, suddenly, without thinking, I vented them. (13m/6)

Can't help laughing, don't know why

After taking the remedy I can't help laughing, don't know why. (12m/2)
In the evening before the oral exam of the doctor's degree I feel agitated, but then I have to have a good laugh about myself and my agitation. (12m/P)

Cries about trivial things

Stuck in a traffic jam. I usually enjoy driving, but today I am close to tears and would really like to just leave the car in the middle of the traffic jam and walk the rest of the way. (4f/2)
I'm constipated. Can't get off to sleep because of the feeling I could explode, and am close to tears. (4f/2)
Impatient, sudden annoyance building up, very easily offended and hurt (could have cried over the most trivial things). (10f/4)

Can't concentrate

Severe rotatory vertigo (something I never get), can't concentrate, can't keep eyes open, improved after lunch. (10f/P)

Confused

Afternoon nap, wake at 3.00 pm and am completely disorientated, can't see what time it is on the clock, still think it is 9.00 am and I should have been at work an hour ago, then become anxious because I've neglected my duty. This lasts for about 2 minutes and only then do I realise that I have

22

only slept for half an hour and that everything is ok. (13m/10P)

Exactly the same situation as on 3.4 [C:even the time is the same] (13m/12P)

<u>Detached</u>

I also feel completely dazed, sometimes don't understand what is going on around me, can't think straight, detached, as if I'm wrapped in cotton wool. (8f/10P)

Dreams

<u>Of animals</u> [14]

I am in my parents' garden .... I come across a badger, large, dangerous, ugly, a cunning face, fast, light brown. It is running around in the garden, then goes through the terrace doors into the building. I can't remember having ever dreamt about animals. It's very strange about the badger. Feeling in the dream: a little frantic, and anxious that the badger could get me, because it moves so quickly and appears in different places all the time. In the dream the animal that I saw looked like a marten, but I knew for sure that it was a badger. (1f/2)

Terrible nightmares that wake me, and continue once I fall back to sleep again. Dreams of dark figures following me; of cats that kill each other and injure each other very severely. The dreams definitely feel very real. (4f/1)

I was on a pond, which consisted more of mud than water. A couple of frogs were sitting in it, croaking peacefully. The strange thing is that at the same time as being a frog myself, I was also observing the scene from outside. All things considered it was a very peaceful atmosphere. (5m/6)

I'm teasing ravens, that are wandering about around me, until they become very angry. They gradually prepare to attack. Just before they attack me I reach a peace settlement with the leader (at the same time I almost don't get away with it, because I'm messing about and and making fun of the situation. (6m/1)

Then I go to the edge of the balcony and look down at the sea. I can see two large rats in the sea and shout to the others how ghastly they are. Suddenly an enormously long, red anaconda surfaces from the depths and everyone, including me, is startled. My mother jumps into the water to take a look at

---

14 In the case of Karl-Josef Müller: Dreams of white ants, of 'big cats', of a wild horse.

them. I shout after her not to do it, but the snake has already encircled her and strangles her. I scream, try to do something and come across a rifle. Nobody else lifts a finger. The snake disappears with my mother into a tunnel, and I shoot after it. The shot causes the snake and tunnel to go up in fire. It is not possible to rescue my mother. I am left with the impression that my mother is still alive, but that tests are going to be carried out on her while she's still inside the snake. At the entrance door where this is taking place I meet 2 friends, also medical students, who are on guard. (6m/15P)

A friend from the past pays a visit to the family home. My young sister is laid up in plaster in her room. I am in my old room from my childhood. My friend stays sitting in the kitchen; my mother is busy cooking, my brothers and sisters are also there; there are cats all over the place; one of the cats falls into the pan that has spinach in it. Then I say that I won't eat at home anymore. The cats are thrown out of the window. (9f/6)

A boy has a small bird perched on his finger. I crouch down next to the boy and the small bird pecks a tick out from my body. (9f/7)

I am playing with the boss's dog, which usually won't allow a living soul close to it. I lie down on a lounger, and in doing so the dog keeps trying to jump up at me. I push him down, he bites my hand. There is no blood visible, my hand hurts tremendously, it feels as if it's been crushed. My boss makes some comment about it. (9f/25P)

<u>Bitten by an animal</u>

I am in my parents' garden .... I come across a badger, large, dangerous, ugly, a cunning face, fast, light brown. It's running around in the garden, then goes through the terrace doors into the building. I try to take a photo of it ... it bites me, digging its teeth into my arm: left arm, the bite is in the dorsal-ulnar in the left wrist, it looks like a small, neat incision, 1/2 cm long, completely smooth, there's hardly any blood coming out of the wound at all. I warn my parents, who are watching television (a current affairs programme) that a badger is in the home. I'm holding my injured arm, I know that it hurts but I don't feel any pain. Dad takes a photograph of the badger. I ask mum for my vaccination certificate to see if I am due to have a tetanus and two additional booster jabs. I think that I am due for one of them. Mum thinks not ... I can't remember having ever dreamt about animals. It's very strange about the badger. Feeling in the dream: a little frantic, and anxious that the badger could get me, because it moves so quickly and appears in different places all the time. In the dream the animal that I saw looked like a marten, but I new for sure that it was a badger. (1f/2)

I am playing with the boss's dog, which usually won't allow a living soul close to it. I lie down on a lounger, and in doing so the dog keeps trying to jump up at me. I push him down, he bites my hand.

24

There is no blood visible, my hand hurts tremendously, it feels as if it's been crushed. My boss makes some comment about it. (9f/25P)

Pursuit - threatened (by a violent woman)

Terrible nightmares that wake me, which continue once I fall back to sleep again. Dreams of dark figures following me, of cats that kill each other and really injure each other severely, and certainly feel the dreams are very realistic. By that I mean that my sleep is very poor, I do not feel at all rested in the morning and then I have to sleep in the daytime, when I don't dream though, but tend to sleep like a log. (4f/1)

Had nightmares again and dreamt about dark figures that were following me; because of that was also extremely frightened of falling asleep; woke once again unrefreshed and had to have a sleep during the day again. (4f/3)

Dreadful dream that was horrifically violent - but also find a solution in the dream and a way to overcome the fear!! There was a lot of detail in the dream and it was very realistic.

I am about to go on a ski course with my class and almost everyone is in the coach. I get out again - there are only a few others outside the coach. Suddenly a woman throws a bomb into the bus and drives away in her car. I memorise the car's registration number and call the police straight away. The police arrive soon after, but say that they can't arrest the woman as they would need a special unit, which they don't have in Austria. Most of the police drive away, only 2 female police, dressed in mini skirts, stay behind - I am frightened, because I know that the woman will be back and there will be no-one to protect me. She actually does come back again and I try to leave discreetly to fetch help, but chat to her so she doesn't catch on that I am aware of who she is. She comes with me and on the way I see some armed men, who are at a wedding/party. I speak to one of the senior men and explain what has happened. He immediately calls for a friend to come along. Feel protected by both of them, although I am still frightened of the woman. I introduce the older man as my grandfather (so that she doesn't become suspicious) and we carry on walking until we come to a kind of children's playground. There is a circle in the middle, in which many people are running.

My 'grandfather' is running with the woman as well. I am with them to begin with, but then become fearful, because, once again, there are so many people in one place and I think she's going to attempt another attack. Which she does. She runs outside of the circle. The first attempt missed the target, which meant that 'my grandfather's' friend can shoot her, but doesn't kill her. Her second attempt is successful and, once again, I am the only survivor. Devastation all around, lots of burnt bodies lying around, the woman walks around and checks whether they are all really dead. I am petrified, pretend to be dead and she doesn't spot me.

25

... I WAKE UP - fall asleep again and carry on dreaming!! (something I never do)

I am living in an apartment very close to where the first attack took place and am worried that she could return. My brother and his wife also live with me. They have moved in on a short-term basis so that I won't be so frightened.

One day I am in a bus and I notice that she is sitting in the bus again. The woman suddenly turns into a man, however, but it takes me a while before I realise this and think 'surely that was a woman before' after which she turns into a woman again. In the meantime I found out that she is having psychotherapy treatment with the sister of a friend of mine, and that the woman sees her attacks as 'school-work' that she has to carry out. (Out of 100 planned mass murders she has only carried out 40!)

I try to make contact with the psychotherapist so that she can talk to the woman. And then it comes to me that in Austria there is WEGA (a police division known for it's brutality) anyway, and they would most definitely be capable of taking her into custody.

... Feel a sense of relief, have much less fear, because I have managed to free myself from this fear and I could protect myself. I can see a way out, was not at all paralysed with fear in the dream as always used to be the case with these kind of nightmares! (8f/26P)

Once again I dream about a violent woman! She is being abusive towards her male friend. On the one hand I am trying to protect him, on the other I am frightened of her and have to protect myself. However, once again I manage to have a talk with her and bring her to her senses. (8f/30P)

Celebrations

The dream consisted of many chaotic sequences and I only remember part of it: There's a New Year's Eve celebration in the building I live in. We have put on a New Year's Eve party in our apartment, which looks totally different in the dream. Even the way in which the other apartments and the corridors are set out is quite different to how they are in reality. Dad - who flew to America to celebrate New Year, and flew straight back - is there. Mum stayed there. New Year is celebrated just one hour earlier than here, how does that equate with the long flight? He's going to fly off somewhere again in the summer. Mum makes some comment about this because she will be on her own. My brother is also there and is running around naked, except for a condom. No-one appears surprised. A friend (Canan) is also there, she had also been to America twice. New neighbours (2 women) have moved in. People from all the other apartments come in and sit by them in my apartment. Chairs are already set out. I think how nice this is to get to know people. These are lots of people that I don't know at all, not the kind of people that actually live in our building. The New Year's Eve party goes on until 3 am, with people celebrating in the whole of the building, many people in the corridors. The next day I get up at 7 am and was thinking I should have stayed on longer. (1f/11P)

I am sitting at a large table, with a group of people who have been invited there to celebrate an occasion: there are people from all over the world, including my parents, and also my brother. (6m/15P)

<u>(Painless) injury to the (left) hand</u>

I am in my parents' garden .... I come across a badger, large, dangerous, ugly, a cunning face, fast, light brown. It is running around in the garden, then goes through the terrace doors into the building. I try to take a photo of it ... it bites me, digging its teeth into my arm: left arm, the bite is in the dorsal-ulnar in the left wrist, it looks like a small, neat incision,_ cm long, completely smooth, the wound is hardly bleeding at all. I have got hold of my injured arm, I know that it hurts but I don't feel any pain. (1f/2)

My mother is driving the car and has to brake hard suddenly. I'm flung out of the car and am thrown quite a distance: beneath me are vines with trellises running parallel and as I'm flying through the air I wonder how my fall is going to be. I try to land causing as little damage as possible, ie I plunge into the vines and brake with my left hand. As I land I notice that I have hardly any injuries, except for a cut on the left hand. They take me to the hospital, my mother is driving too slowly, and very badly. My father is sitting in the back, pretty annoyed with her and wants to take over the driving. (6m/19P)

I am playing with the boss's dog, which usually won't allow a living soul close to it. I lie down on a lounger, and in doing so the dog keeps trying to jump up at me. I push him down, he bites me on hand. There is no blood visible, my hand hurts tremendously, it feels as if it's been crushed. My boss makes some comment about it. (9f/25P)

<u>Frantic, chaotic</u> [15]

Feeling in the dream: a little frantic and anxious that the badger could get me, because it moves so quickly and is constantly in a different place. (1f/2)

The whole of the time I have the feeling that I have to 'escape' to my room, before my dad sees me. I feel frantic inside. Her mustn't see me. It's absolutely okay for my brother and my mum to see me, and they do, and it's also totally okay for me to be in the kitchen. The whole of the time I'm just

---

[15] Confirmed several times by K.-J. Müllers proving.

frightened that dad will see me. This frantic feeling runs through the whole dream. The dream ends as I want to go back into my room again. (1f/7P)

The dream consisted of many muddled sequences and I only remembered part of it. (1f/11P)

<u>Relatives</u>

I am in my parent's garden ... Mum had been weeding ... I warn my parents, who are watching television (a current affairs programme), there's a badger inside ... dad takes a photograph of the badger. I ask mum for my vaccination certificate. (1f/2)

I am still living at home with my parents. I come down from my room (on the 1st floor) into the kitchen, and take muesli and milk from the fridge. The muesli and milk are in a white bowl with a golden rim. I have to heat up the milk in the microwave. To do this I have to empty it into a different container that doesn't have a gold rim. I tip it out a couple of times until everything is just right, because on a couple of occasions I spilt some. In the end I've got two warmed up bowls with golden rims containing milk and muesli. While this has been going on my brother and parents are sitting in the living room. The whole of the time I have the feeling that I will have to 'escape' again to my room before my dad sees me. I feel frantic inside. He mustn't see me. It's absolutely okay for my brother and my mum to see me, and they do, and it's also totally okay for me to be in the kitchen. All the time I'm just frightened that dad will see me. This frantic feeling runs through the whole dream. The dream ends as I want to go back into my room again. (1f/7P)

I have noticed that the badger dream also took place in my parents' home and that in both dreams I was still living in the family home, and not just there for a visit. (I have been living in my own apartment for the last 1 _ years). In the dreams the rooms looked identical to how they are in real life. (1f/P)

I don't usually have nightmares: I fell asleep and began to feel frightened that I wouldn't be able to control my thoughts. I went through the dark apartment and woke my mother. Light improved the situation and my thoughts came to a halt. (6m/9)

I am sitting at a large table, with a group of people who have been invited there to celebrate an occasion: there are people from all over the world, including my parents, and also my brother.... (6m/15P)

Then I go to the edge of the balcony and look down at the sea. I can see two large rats in the sea and shout to the others how ghastly they are. Suddenly an enormously long, red anaconda surfaces from the depths and everyone, including me, is startled. My mother jumps into the water to take a look at them. I shout after her not to do it, but the snake has already encircled her and strangles her. I scream, try to do something and come across a rifle. Nobody else lifts a finger. The snake disappears with my mother into a tunnel, and I shoot after it. The shot causes the snake and tunnel to go up in fire. It is not possible to rescue my mother. I am left with the impression that my mother is still alive, but that tests are going to be carried out on her while she's still inside the snake. At the entrance door where this is taking place I meet 2 friends, also medical students, who are on guard. (6m/15P)

My mother is driving the car and has to brake hard suddenly. I'm flung out of the car and am thrown quite a distance: beneath me are vines with trellises running parallel and as I'm flying through the air I wonder how my fall is going to be. I try to land causing as little damage as possible, i.e. I plunge into the vines and brake with my left hand. As I land I notice that I have hardly any injuries, except for a cut on the left hand. They take me to the hospital, my mother is driving too slowly, and very badly. My father is sitting in the back, pretty annoyed with her and wants to take over the driving. (6m/19P)

My sister is at home with her leg in plaster. She has something between a plaster, which allows the patient to walk, and one that restricts the patient from moving about.

A friend from the past pays a visit to the family home. My young sister is laid up in plaster in her room. I am in my old room from my childhood. My friend stays sitting in the kitchen; my mother is busy cooking, my brothers and sisters are also there; there are cats all over the place; one of the cats falls into the pan with spinach in. Then I say that I won't eat at home anymore. The cats are thrown out of the window. (9f/6)

Sweets

And the yearning for sweet things is still there! And follows me into my sleep, and I dream about vanilla croissants and other sweet things, so that I wake up in the morning with incredible hunger and can't stop thinking about sweet things the whole day. This improves when I eat something sweet. (4f/3)

(Explosive) weapons

Suddenly a woman throws a bomb into the coach and drives away in her car ...
On the way I see some armed men, who are at a wedding/party. I speak to a senior man and explain what has happened. He immediately calls for a friend to come along. Feel protected by both of them although I am still frightened of the woman... We carry on walking to a kind of children's playground. There is a circle in the middle, in which many people are running. My 'grandfather' is running with the woman as well. I am with them to begin with, but then become fearful, because once again there are so many people in one place and I think that she's going to attempt another

attack. Which she does. She runs outside the circle, the first attempt missed the target, so that 'my grandfather's' friend can shoot her, but doesn't kill her. Her second attempt is successful and I am the only survivor once again. Devastation all around, lots of burnt bodies lying around, the woman walks around and checks whether they are all really dead, I am petrified, pretend to be dead and she doesn't spot me ... In the meantime I have found out that she is having psychotherapy treatment with the sister of a friend of mine, and that the woman sees her attacks as 'school-work' that she has to carry out. (out of 100 planned mass murders she has only carried out 40 !) (8f/26P)

Vertigo

Vertigo, 'Queasy', muzzy - and dead tired with it

Feel dizzy and sometimes feel like the earth is swaying under me. When I fix my gaze on an object it starts to move. I have a lie- down in bed again at lunchtime, take a while to get warm and am completely worn out. When I stand up I feel very dizzy again. When I stand up quickly, everything turns black. I feel better into the afternoon and evening. (8f/9P)
Get up in the morning as usual and feel well to begin with - but then the dizziness starts again. I also feel completely dazed, sometimes don't understand what is going on around me, can't think straight, detached, as if I'm wrapped in cotton wool. Go back to bed again at midday, completely worn out. (8f/10P)
Slight dizziness and a bit shaky at approximately 11.00am, with weakness and the need to eat something immediately to relieve these symptoms. (9f/6)
Slight dizziness again in the morning, a bit shaky, nervous, jittery, like I'd drunk too much strong black tee - revved up. Legs somewhat weak.
Increased weakness when walking fast, dizziness. (9f/8)
Somewhat nervous, jittery, dizzy and nauseous (as if I'd have to be sick) after enjoying half a litre of green tea around 10.00 am.
A mild, dull headache in the temples after a walk at 12.00 midday, weakness and again the feeling that this weakness could be remedied by eating (But I just ate beforehand.) (9f/16P)
Around 4.00 pm mild headache in the temples again, mild dizziness. Lasts until around 5.00 pm. (9f/28P)
Severe rotatory vertigo (something I never get). (10f/P)

Detached, wrapped in cotton wool

Get up in the morning as usual and feel well to begin with - but then the dizziness starts again. I also feel completely dazed, sometimes don't understand what is going on around me, can't think straight, detached, as if I'm wrapped in cotton wool. Go back to bed again at midday, completely worn out. (8f/10P)

30

Rotatory vertigo

Severe rotatory vertigo (something I never get). (10f/P)

Vertigo when standing up suddenly; when walking fast

When I stand up I feel dizzy again. When I stand up quickly everything turns black. I feel better into the afternoon and evening. (8f/9P)
Increased weakness when walking fast, dizziness. (9f/8)

Balance is not as good during yoga

Balance is not as good during yoga. (11f/4)

Earth is swaying, objects move when fixing gaze on them, the wall is closing in on me

Feel dizzy and sometimes feel like the earth is swaying under me. When I fix my gaze on an object it starts to move. (8f/9P)
While sitting I suddenly have the feeling as if the wall to the right of me was moving towards me. (8f/20P)

Headache

I got a headache on the 5th day. But totally different to the ones I'm used to. It started in the morning after waking (but I didn't wake up because of it), increasing in strength as the morning progressed and was gone after lunch. Mild in intensity; located in the occiput, radiating to the neck and both temples, just under the scalp. I can't answer the question as to 'how' it is. It felt similar to after having slept in the wrong position, making my head and neck stiff in the morning. Better: Sitting, distraction, ascending stairs. Worse: Walking straight ahead. (1f/5P)
Mild headache in the afternoon (around the frontal sinuses). (2f/1)
From midday superficial headache (left sided neuralgia; two cervical vertebrae were released the day before - is there a connection? (2f/7)
Head symptoms as the previous day, increasing tendency towards extreme tension in the trapezius. (2f/8)
From midday onwards some tension headache, eases about an hour after finishing work. (2f/23P)
Despite sleeping for a long time I am still very tired and worn out, and later on I have a headache (right temple, pulsating pain, better from pressure and massaging neck/upper back). (8f/24P)

Mild, dull headache in the temples until around 3.00 pm. (9f/6)

Mild, dull headache at 12.00 midday after a walk. (9f/16P)

At 4.00 pm mild headache in the temples again. (9w/19N)

Mild pain in the temples at midday. Pains increase somewhat in the fresh air - mild breeze - while walking.

More severe headache at 3.00 pm, feeling my head will explode when bending down. The pains last until I go to bed. (9f/21P)

Mild headache again in the morning, as yesterday. Gone by midday. (9f/22P)

Stabbing yet bearable headache in the area to the left at the back (around the petrous bone), in the late afternoon. (12m/1)

Pain in various parts of the body, come and go very quickly e.g. headache left temple for approximately _ seconds, like stabbing or an electric shock. (13m/6)

Headache from midday onwards: Forehead, throbbing, more to the left. Worse from motion; bending down increases the pain. In the afternoon (approximately 4.00 pm) a pressing pain in the head, from the sides inwards, stronger on the left. No headache the following morning (unusual: usually the headache is still there in the morning). (14f/4)

Mild headache again from midday : throbbing, pulsating, stronger on the right side; more severe in the evenings again; gone by the following morning. (14f/5)

Pressure behind the eyes, mild frontal headache, irrespective of body position. (15f/1)

Headache is of no consequence now. (15f/2)

Headache is temporal at this point in time [C: 5.00-8.00 pm], on both sides. Ameliorated by running. (15f/15)

In the temples

Despite sleeping for a long time I am still very tired and worn out, and later on I have a headache (right temple, pulsating pain, better from pressure and massaging neck/upper back). (8f/24P)

Mild, dull headache in the temples until around 3.00 pm. (9f/6)

A mild, dull headache in the temples after a walk at 12.00 midday. (9f/16P)

At 4.00 pm mild headache in the temples again. (9f/19P)

Mild pain in the temples at midday. Pains increase somewhat in the fresh air - mild breeze - while walking.

More severe headache at 3.00 pm, feeling my head will explode when bending down. The pains last until I go to bed. (9f/21P)

Mild headache again in the morning, as yesterday. Gone by midday. (9f/22P)

Pain in various parts of the body, come and go very quickly e.g. headache left temple for approximately _ seconds, like stabbing or an electric shock. (13m/6)

Headache is temporal at this point in time [C: 5.00-8.00 pm], on both sides. Ameliorated by running. (15f/15)

Face, Eye, Ear

Red face

Face as red as a beetroot after the gym, particularly the cheeks (this is normal), but this reddening of the face goes on for hours on end. When touching the cheeks the skin feels sore, burning, hot, like sunburn. (1f/14P)

Dry Lips

My lips are very dry, rough and split easy. They are no better after lubricating them. (8f/6P)
Lips become even more raw, sore, feel split. (8f/7P)
Lips are not improving, and now also a mild rash around the lips, small dots, reddish, which are already apparent from a distance. Particularly around the corner of the mouth. (8f/9P)

(Rash around the) Eyes

For a long time my skin eruptions have been very intense again generally - particularly very painful on the eyelids. (8f/24P)
Small rash under the eyes (particularly the left) - small red spots on rising. (10f/2)
Eyes feel stuck together. | (10f/approx. 30P)
Slightly swollen eyes in the morning. (15f/11)

Stabbing in the ears

Brief, mild stabbing pain, alternating between left and right ear, with long intervals in-between. (2f/2)
A stabbing pain in the ears, which came on straight away, on the way home after a swim at the baths - alternating left and right (I never get this usually). (10f/25P)
Since then, symptoms for over a week again, particularly evenings ... occasional stabbing in the ears, particularly during the day. (10f/approx.30P)
(After consultation) antidoted with a single dose of Sepia Q5 [C: because of toothache].
Earache still from time to time since then, lasting a short time. (10f/approx.40P)

Mouth and Throat

Sore areas on the roof of the mouth, open, 'raw' mucous membranes in mouth and lips, apthae.

Small cold sore inside the right cheek in the evening. (2f/13)
Since today I have a sore spot on the roof of the mouth, just behind the incisors at the side. This area burns and feels extremely unpleasant when I'm eating. (4f/3)
And the sore patch on the roof of the mouth is also still there. (4f/4)
The sore spot on the roof of the mouth is still there. (4f/5)
The sore spot on the roof of the mouth is also still there. It itches and is painful. (4f/6)
The sore spot on the roof of the mouth is still there. (4f/7)
The sore spot on the roof of the mouth cleared up immediately as soon as I stopped taking the globules. (4f/P)
Early in the morning, pain in the mucous membranes in my mouth and an exposed feeling (right interior upper lip). I can see a small light, blister. (8f/4)

Bright red margin around the teeth

Dentist appointment - bright red margin around the gums, especially lower jaw, as if swollen, gingiva is usually very pale - otherwise teeth are okay, no leaky fillings. (10f/6P)
Dental problems only occasionally in the evenings. The margin around the teeth is becoming distinctly paler (although still visible). (10f/25P)

Dry mouth and throat with unquenchable thirst

Throughout the whole day I have really extreme, almost unquenchable, thirst and also an extremely dry throat. (4f/2)
Once again I have an almost unquenchable thirst and an extremely dry throat which lasts the whole day. (4f/3)
Extreme thirst and a dry throat. (4f/4)
Extreme thirst and a dry throat. (4f/5)
I still have great thirst and in the afternoon I was out and about and suddenly really felt like I was going to die of thirst, it was particularly strong. I had to buy something to drink immediately as my throat was totally parched. My thoughts were revolving around getting something to drink and I couldn't get rid of them until I had drunk something. This is how it must feel in the desert!! (4f/6)
Very dry sensation in the mouth, great thirst (more than usual). (10f/1)
Very parched. (10f/2)
Small amount of urine (despite drinking a lot), extremely dried up (particularly the mouth; a feeling as if my tongue is swelling up. (10f/3)

Noticeably dry mouth during work out on the exercise bike in the gym. (15f/7).
Feel very well, dry mouth again during work-out. (15f/8)
Good general state of health, despite little sleep. still have a rather dry mouth. (15f/13)

Heartburn

Heartburn after eating chilli (never have usually). (13m/9P)

Bad breath

I am aware of a particularly 'noxious' mouth odour in the morning on waking. (1f/8-16P)

Teeth

Toothache, as if food was trapped

Beginning of the toothache - Sensation as if food was trapped in the bottom left side of the mouth (which was not the case however). Later this unpleasant sensation also extended out to the front upper jawbone. In various parts of the mouth I had the sensation as if the teeth were loose, particularly as I was falling asleep, or once I woke up in the night I was unable to fall asleep again. (10f/5)
Toothache is better (the sensation of having to bite on something has improved). There is only discomfort in the bottom left hand side.
Dentist appointment - bright red margin around the gums, especially lower jaw, as if swollen, gingiva is usually very pale - otherwise teeth are okay, no leaky fillings. (10f/6P)
Toothache continues, particularly at night; relatively pain-free during the day. Sensation of food trapped for a while again in the evening, better from eating. (10f/7-12P)
Dental problems only occasionally in the evenings. The margin around the teeth is becoming distinctly paler (although still visible). (10f/25P)
Went to the swimming baths - in the evening this unpleasant toothache again, particularly on the left hand lower side again; feeling that something is twinging. (10f/27P)
Antidoted with a single dose of Sepia Q5 (after a consultation) - the toothache actually disappeared on the same day.
Took Sepia Q5 again (a week later) after another episode of toothache. (10f/approx. 40P)

Teeth feel loose, better for clenching them

Beginning of the toothache ... alternating between various parts of the mouth I had a sensation as if the teeth were coming loose, particularly as I was falling asleep, or rather once I woke up in the night

35

I was unable to fall asleep again. (10f/5)
Toothache, feel I need to clench my teeth, which helps. (10f/6P)

Sensations in the teeth

Teeth are becoming a topic. No pain, more like mouth currents or a pulling sensation, most noticeable on the upper jaw. (15f/22P)
Conscious of the teeth in a strange way, up to the roots. (15f/23P)
Conscious of all my teeth from time to time, no pain. Especially evenings. (15f/24P)

Stomach

Heartburn

Heartburn after eating chilli (never have usually). (13m/9P)

Unquenchable thirst with dry mouth and throat

Throughout the whole day I have really extreme, almost unquenchable, thirst and also an extremely dry throat. (4f/2)
Once again I have an almost unquenchable thirst and an extremely dry throat which lasts the whole of the day. (4f/3)
Extreme thirst and a dry throat (4f/4)
Extreme thirst and a dry throat. (4f/5)
I still have great thirst and in the afternoon I was out and about and suddenly really felt like I was going to die of thirst, it was particularly strong. I had to buy something to drink immediately as my throat was totally parched. My thoughts were revolving around getting something to drink and I couldn't get rid of them until I had drunk something. This is how it must feel in the desert!! (4f/6)
Very dry sensation in the mouth, great thirst (more than usual). (10f/1)
Very dry mouth still and constant thirst. (10m/25P)

Thirst for cold drinks

I quenched my thirst with cold drinks, tending towards water, or mineral water. The desire for cold drinks was definitely greater than for warm (although I tend to be more of a tea drinker usually and drink a lot of tea during the day!). (4m/P)

Abdomen

Meteorism, 'Knot in abdomen'

My bowels are rebelling ie I am constipated, and when I lie down to go to sleep in the evening all my thoughts revolve around my bowels and it feels that somehow there is a knot in there. Can hardly fall asleep as I feel like I'm going to explode, and am close to tears. Then I put a hot water bottle on my abdomen, which relieves a little. (4f/2)
I am still constipated and my abdomen is distended as well. (4f/3)
I continue to have a distended abdomen and am still constipated. (4f/4)
I also continue to be constipated and have a distended abdomen. (4f/5)
And I am also still constipated and full of wind. (4f/6)
The sore spot on the roof of the mouth cleared up immediately as soon as I stopped taking the globules. But I am still constipated and full of wind. And this desire for sweets and the terrible thirst has returned to normal. (4f/P)
Meteorism again. (10f/3)
Slight sensation of lead in the abdomen. (11f/5)
The sensation of 'lead belly' and meteorism again in the evening. (11f/8)

Rectum

Foul smelling flatulence

From today, severe, strong-smelling flatulence, lasting a few days. (2f/18)
My bowels are rebelling ie I am constipated, and when I lie down to go to sleep in the evening all my thoughts revolve around my bowels and it feels that somehow there is a knot in there. Can hardly fall asleep as I feel like I'm going to explode, and am close to tears. Then I put a hot water bottle on my abdomen, which relieves a little. (4f/2)
I am still constipated and my abdomen is distended as well. (4f/3)
I continue to have a distended abdomen and am still constipated. (4f/4)
I also continue to be constipated and have a distended abdomen. (4f/5)
And I am also still constipated and full of wind. (4f/6)
The sore spot on the roof of the mouth cleared up immediately as soon as I stopped taking the globuli. But I am am still constipated and full of wind. And this desire for sweets and the terrible thirst has returned to normal. (4f/P)
Considerable flatulence, loud and extremely foul-smelling, which began in the afternoon and was worse in the evenings. (13m/3)
Flatulence has gone in the morning, appearing again in the afternoon, and at it's worst in the evenings. (13m/4)

Flatulence as above, worse after eating and evenings, better in the morning. (13m/5)
Still have flatulence. (13m/6)
Flatulence subsiding. (13m/8P)

<u>Constipated</u>

My bowels are rebelling i.e. I am constipated, and when I lie down to go to sleep in the evening all my thoughts revolve around my bowels and it feels that somehow there is a knot in there. Can hardly fall asleep as I feel like I'm going to explode, and am close to tears. Then I put a hot water bottle on my abdomen, which relieves a little. (4f/2)
I am still constipated and my abdomen is distended as well. (4f/3)
I also continue to be constipated and have a distended abdomen. (4f/5)
And I am also still constipated and full of wind. (4f/6)
The sore spot on the roof of the mouth cleared up immediately as soon as I stopped taking the globuli. But I am am still constipated and full of wind. And this desire for sweets and the terrible thirst has returned to normal. (4f/P)

<u>Foul-smelling stool</u>

My stool has a similar 'noxious', pungent, odour [C: as mouth odour]. (1f/10-14P)

Female genitalia

<u>Menses too early.</u>

Menses in the morning - a week too soon! (11f/12P)

<u>Menses too late</u>

My cycle is never spot-on, usually a couple of days late, but this time it was 36 days (oligomenorrhoea), which is, however, distinctly longer than normal. Besides this, there are a couple of additional reasons that have me convinced that the remedy is responsible for the delay: Sometimes I get a fungal infection on the vulva a couple of days before my period, which lasts until the first or second day of my period. I also got it this time, on time, and it lasted as long as usual and then subsided, without my period having started. From the 10th day both breasts were feeling swollen and sensitive to pressure (I never have this otherwise), continuing until the last day of my period. (1f)

Painful periods (dysmenorrhoea)

Feel a light to medium dragging sensation in right lower abdomen, at the build-up to my period. Sensation as if everything had cramped up inside my lower abdomen.

Sensitive to pressure, better for warmth, as also curling up into a ball/squatting.

Haven't had pain like this for a long time, and would only get it during the day, never at night when I'm lying in bed!

This time I even wake in the night and lie awake for a while in pain.

Pain is a bit better first thing in the morning (at other times it was the exact opposite), but time and time again intense dragging and cramps, that come on suddenly, in the whole of the lower abdomen. No longer any pain in the late afternoon and evening. (8f)

Breast

Mammae

From the 10th day [C: of the cycle] *both breasts were feeling swollen and sensitive to pressure (I never have this otherwise), continuing until the last day of my period.* (1f)

Extremities

Warm, foul-smelling foot sweat

I already noticed increased perspiration on both feet on the first day of taking the remedy. Usually in the wintertime I often wear 2 pairs of socks at home, a pair of thin and a pair of thick, hand-knitted woollen socks (instead of slippers). On the 2nd day I manage with a pair of thin socks. By the 4th day the 'sweaty feet' have taken shape quite distinctly. On the 4th day I don't feel I need to have any socks on at all, but put on a pair of thin ones anyway. Usually, from time to time, I also put on a pair of thin socks in the night, and now don't need to do that at all any more. Usually I can wear the same socks for a couple of days, and then only wash them because it occurs to me I've had them on a while, not because they are sweaty. Now I change my socks every day. The soles of my feet are always somewhat damp and smell slightly similar to Gouda cheese. The perspiration does not damage the skin, there is no discolouration. It's very embarrassing for me if I'm invited somewhere where I have to take my shoes off. I hope people can't smell my feet. On the 4th day I went for a walk in the evening wearing casual shoes. It was particularly cool; usually my toes would be extremely cold when I get home. Instead they are sweaty today, my socks are so damp that I can see my footprints on the floor. The damp areas are where the shoe was covering the feet. When I touch my feet they feel cold and damp and a little spongy. Over the next few days I also sweat more in the evenings when I take a walk than when I am at home in the daytime. My feet do not sweat when I have no socks on. The foot sweat subsided again from the 10th day and decreases as the days go by, until it disappeared completely on the 17th day. (1f/1-17P)

<u>Pain in the shoulder [16] (left)</u>

Distinct decrease in the pains in my shoulder. (11f/1)
Continued decrease in the pain in my left shoulder. (11f/2)
Around 80% improvement in the shoulder. (11f/5)
Except for an increase in shoulder pain, no distinguishing symptoms or distinctive features over the next days, as before taking the remedy ... Would like it best if I could carry on taking the remedy. (11f/18P)

Chill

<u>Feeling cold, extreme at the present time - mornings on waking - in the early morning hours</u>

The sensitivity to cold from the previous days continues (viral infection?). Better after spicy food at midday (blood pressure?). (2f/1)
Feeling cold just before getting up, in spite of a duvet. (2f/5)
Feeling extremely cold in the morning. It feels like I'm not covered up, lasting approximately 45 minutes - takes a long time for me to get warm. Later on I realise that I already had this chilly feeling in the morning a week ago, but less marked. (2f/13)
Cold in bed during the night. (11f/1)
In the evening before falling asleep feel very cold in bed again. (11f/2)
Feel cold, have a hot bath in the evening. (11f/11P)
Extremely tired and worn out in the afternoon, went to bed, frozen and tired out. (15f/1)
Still occasional shivering, particularly in the morning. (15f/2)
Felt frozen in the night despite being wrapped up warm. (15f/3)

16
    K.-J. Müller's proving : *crushed* feeling in the shoulders, and cramping pains in the shoulder in another prover

Feeling cold in the morning for a short time. (15f/6)
Very cold in the afternoon. (15f/13)
Frozen during the night despite a warm duvet. (15f/14)
Retrospective comment: The cold feeling that I experienced during the proving was completely new for me, and it hasn't happened again since then. I would wake up in the early hours because I felt cold, and also felt chilly around 4 pm and couldn't get warm. There are no symptoms left over from the proving, I feel very well and the ups and downs in terms of energy, from during the proving, are now over. (15f/P)

Feeling cold in bed

Feeling cold just before getting up, in spite of a duvet. (2f/5)
No feeling cold in the night anymore. (2f/6)
Cold in bed during the night. (11f/1)
In the evening before falling asleep feel very cold in bed again. (11f/2)
Felt frozen in the night despite being wrapped up warm. (15f/3)
Frozen during the night despite a warm duvet. (15f/14)
I woke up in the early hours because I felt cold. (15f/P)

Can't get warm

I woke up in the early hours because I felt cold, and also felt chilly around 4 pm and couldn't get warm. (15f/P)

Perspiration

Night sweats

No night sweats anymore (used to get them often in the past - after the baby was born in July 2000). (10f/2)
Slight night sweat. (11f/8)
Disturbed sleep, profuse night sweat again. My nightie was completely soaked! (11f/9)
Profuse night sweat, especially axillae. (11f/11P)

(Dream that) back is sweating

Dream: On the way back I notice that I am sweating on the upper part of my body, but it also doesn't really bother me (in front of the others). (6m/18P)

Warm, foul-smelling foot sweat

I already noticed increased perspiration on both feet on the first day of taking the remedy. Usually in the wintertime I often wear 2 pairs of socks at home, a pair of thin and a pair of thick, hand-knitted woollen socks (instead of slippers). On the 2nd day I manage with a pair of thin socks. By the 4th day the 'sweaty feet' have taken shape quite distinctly. On the 4th day I don't feel I need to have any socks on at all, but put on a pair of thin ones anyway. Usually, from time to time, I also put on a pair of thin socks in the night, and now don't need to do that at all any more. Usually I can wear the same socks for a couple of days, and then only wash them because it occurs to me I've had them on a while, not because they are sweaty. Now I change my socks every day. The soles of my feet are always somewhat damp and smell slightly similar to Gouda cheese. The perspiration does not damage the skin, there is no discolouration. It's very embarrassing for me if I'm invited somewhere where I have to take my shoes off. I hope people can't smell my feet. On the 4th day I went for a walk in the evening wearing casual shoes. It was particularly cool; usually my toes would be extremely cold when I get home. Instead they are sweaty today, my socks are so damp that I can see my footprints on the floor. The damp areas are where the shoe was covering the feet. When I touch my feet they feel cold and damp and a little spongy. Over the next few days I also sweat more in the evenings when I take a walk than when I am at home in the daytime. My feet do not sweat when I have no socks on. The foot sweat subsided again from the 10th day and decreases as the days go by, until it disappeared completely on the 17th day. (1f/1-17P)

Generalities

Symptoms that appear (and disappear) suddenly

At midday sudden, stabbing pain in right upper abdomen, can hardly move, only bearable lying quietly on my back, aggravated by movement (including breathing), accompanied by mild nausea, go to the toilet - immediate improvement, no longer any pain. (8f/9P)
A stabbing pain in left elbow joint came on suddenly in the afternoon. The pain comes on when I move a certain way, then stops again suddenly - spreading to the wrist. Later on also a pain in the coccyx area, same modality. (8f/19P)
Time and time again intense dragging and cramps in the whole lower abdomen that come on suddenly [C· during menses]. (8f)
Dull pain in left forearm, radiating, came and went quickly. (13m/5)
Pain in various parts of the body, come and go very quickly e.g. headache left temple for approximately _ seconds, like stabbing or an electric shock. (13m/6)

42

Symptoms changing location (suddenly)

Brief, mild stabbing pain, alternating between left and right ear, with long intervals in-between. (2f/2)

A stabbing pain in the ears, which came on straight away, on the way home after a swim at the baths - alternating left and right (I never get this usually). (10f/25P)

Alternating between various parts of the mouth I had the sensation as if the teeth were loose, particularly as I was falling asleep, or once I woke up in the night I was unable to fall asleep again. (10f/5)

A stabbing pain in the ears, which came on straight away, on the way home after a swim at the baths - alternating left and right (I never get this usually). (10f/25P)

Dull pain in left forearm, radiating, came and went quickly. Pain then moved very quickly to the right occiput and then disappeared (approximately 4.30 pm). Not affected by motion, pressure or warmth (13m/5)

Pain in various parts of the body, come and go very quickly e.g. headache left temple for approximately _ seconds, like stabbing or an electric shock. (13m/6)

Left side

From midday superficial headache (left sided neuralgia; two cervical vertebrae were worked on the day before - is there a connection? (2f/7)

Nothing noteworthy, tension in the left trapezius in the evening again. (2f/15)

Small rash under the eyes (particularly the left) - small red spots on rising. (10f/2)

Sensation as if food was trapped in the bottom left side of the mouth (which was not the case however). (10f/5)

A stabbing pain in left elbow joint came on suddenly in the afternoon. The pain comes on when I move a certain way, then stops again suddenly - spreading to the wrist. (8f/19P)

This unpleasant toothache again in the evening, particularly left side underneath again. (10f/25P)

Decrease in the pain in my left shoulder. (11f/2)

Headache from midday, forehead, throbbing, more on the left, worse for motion, bending down increases the pain.

Headache from midday onwards: Forehead, throbbing, more to the left. Worse from motion; bending down increases the pain. In the afternoon (approximately 4.00 pm) a pressing pain in the head, from the sides inwards, stronger on the left. No headache the following morning (unusual: usually the headache is still there in the morning). (14f/4)

Right side

Right-sided inflammation:

1] Day 5: *on the right big toe the nail is growing inward, pus is building up.*

Around the ingrown nail the area of the toe is red, swollen and painful. This is something I get from time to time, but this time it has lasted a lot longer than usual, up to 17 days, although the toe was not suppurating all this time. The pain was on its way out by the 13th day and a callus had formed. On the 17th day I cut as much of the nail away as possible; the pain stopped from this moment on and the inflammation disappeared completely.

2] Day 9: Since this evening the middle part of my right upper lid, about 1/3rd of the upper lid, has been swollen and red and hurts a bit. On day 11 it is at it's worst, somewhat improved when I run cold water over it or put a cold, damp cloth on it. On day 12 I notice that the pain has completely disappeared, after going for a jog and a shower (not sure what caused it disappear - cool air, motion or the warm water) But the redness and swelling carried on until day 15.

3] Day 9: I have found a small, inflamed spot, red and painful on the right buttock, which lasted some days.

4] Day 10: The nail wall is suppurating on the right middle finger, as if I had pulled the nail back (which I have not) and it had grown into the flesh. The lesion is painful, red and swollen until day 15. (1f)

Early in the morning pain in the mucous membranes in my mouth and an exposed feeling (right interior upper lip). I can see a small light, blister. (8f/4)

Wake up with a sore throat, right side. Feel as if inhaling cold air when breathing through the right nostril. (8f/6P)

While sitting I suddenly have the feeling as if the wall to the right of me was moving towards me. (8f/20P)

Despite sleeping for a long time I am still very tired and worn out, and later on I get a headache (right temple, pulsating pain, better from pressure and massaging neck/upper back). (8f/24P)

Mild headache again from midday : throbbing, pulsating, stronger on the right side; more severe in the evenings again; gone by the following morning. (14f/5)

Today I am aware of recurring pains in the right hip of a pre-arthritic character. (15f/16)

Alternating sides

Brief and mild, stabbing pain alternating between left then right ear, with large intervals in-between. (2f/1)

A stabbing pain in the ears, which came on straight away, on the way home after a swim at the baths - alternating left and right (I never get this usually). (10f/25P)

Offensive secretions

I am aware of a particularly 'noxious' mouth odour in the morning on waking. (1f/8-16P)

My stool has a similar 'noxious', pungent, odour [C.: as mouth odour]. (1f/10-14P)

From today, severe, strong-smelling flatulence, lasting a few days (2f/18)

Considerable flatulence, loud and extremely foul-smelling, which began in the afternoon and was worse in the evenings. (13m/3)

Flatulence has gone in the morning, appearing again in the afternoon, and at it's worst in the evenings. (13m/4)

Flatulence as above, worse after eating and evenings, better in the morning. (13m/5)

Still have flatulence. (13m/6)

Flatulence subsiding. (13m/8P)

I already noticed increased perspiration on both feet on the first day of taking the remedy... By the 4th day the 'sweaty feet' have taken shape quite distinctly... The soles of my feet are always somewhat damp and smell slightly similar to Gouda cheese. The perspiration does not damage the skin, there is no discolouration. It's very embarrassing for me if I am invited somewhere where I have to take my shoes off, I think hopefully people can't smell my feet. (1f/1-17P)

Desire for (soft) sweet food

Standing at the sausage counter and can't make up my mind what to have to eat, and then decide on a 'Wurstsemmel' (sliced sausage in a roll) and as soon as I've got it in my hand I realise that I actually don't fancy it. I eat it nevertheless and realise that I absolutely loathe the sausage meat. I would have actually really preferred to have had something sweet. (4f/2)

Even though I'm not hungry I also constantly feel I need to eat something sweet, and am happy and content if I can have some toast and jam, and somehow not satisfied if I eat sliced sausage on bread or a veal cutlet. (4f/2)

And the yearning for sweet things is still there! And follows me into my sleep, and I dream about vanilla croissants and other sweet things, so that I wake up in the morning with incredible hunger and can't stop thinking about sweet things the whole day. This improves when I eat something sweet. (4f/3)

Craving for sweet food, almost constant; but I'm not prepared to go and buy some ice-cream or something. Instead I pester my brother to go and am then pretty annoyed when he doesn't go. But the craving for sweet things - strangely enough, only for cakes or tiramisu, ie soft desserts - blocks my thoughts completely. (4f/4)

Still have a craving for sweet things. (4f/5)

After eating an enormous amount of sweet things yesterday the craving is not so strong today. (4f/6)

The desire for sweet things has now gone, at last. (4f/7)

Aversion / sensitivity to coffee

'Lead belly' at lunchtime after coffee. (11f/4)

Sudden aversion to coffee. (15f/2)

Aversion to coffee continues. (15f/3)

Pain in lower abdomen, better in the evening, aversion to coffee. (15f/4)

Seems I can smell coffee in the morning, without any reason. (15f/11)

<u>Desire for tea</u>

Developed a liking for tea. (11f/7)
Continue to have a liking for tea (am more of a coffee drinker). (11f/8)

<u>Desire for cold drinks</u>

I quenched my thirst with cold drinks, tending towards water, or mineral water. The desire for cold drinks was definitely greater than for warm (although I tend to be more of a tea drinker usually and drink a lot of tea during the day!). (4f/P)

Energy

<u>Tiredness (evenings) - heavy as lead</u>

Very tired during the day. (2f/1)
Pretty tired since the last few days. (2f/2)
Very tired, not able to do much. (2f/10)
Above all feeling tired in the morning (blood pressure?) (2f/11)
Tiredness, as heavy as lead; exhaustion, especially from late afternoon until evening. (2f/13)
Really tired in the evening. (2f/16)
Very tired from the morning onwards, lasting the whole day. (2f/17)
Extremely intense tiredness in the evening. (3m/7)
All of a sudden very tired and grumpy in the afternoon. Feel completely shattered and worn out, don't feel like doing anything, everything and everyone is getting on my nerves. (8f/3)
Have a lie down in bed at midday, take a while to get warm, feel dead tired. (8f/9P)
Have a lie down in bed at midday, dead tired. (8f/10P)
Despite sleeping for a long time I am still very tired and worn out. (8f/24P)
Am very tired and worn out. (8f/34P)
Felt very tired, 'done-in', went to bed early. (10f/2)
Tiredness in the afternoon - slept for 4 hours. (11f/1)
Great tiredness in the afternoon. (11f/14P)
Extremely tired and exhausted in the afternoon. Went to bed, frozen and sleepy.
On getting up felt exhausted. Better from eating in the evening. (15f/1)
Very tired. (15f/2)
Tired, but not exhausted. (15f/3)
Mentally and physically able, although continue to be tired. (15f/4)

46

Very tired, not able to do much. (15f/10)
Extremely tired, better from midday. (15f/11)
Tired more in the afternoon. (15f/14)
Feel like I've not had enough sleep in the morning, despite sleeping until 10.00 am. (11.00 am) (15f/P)

Tired, but can't fall asleep

Unusually intense tiredness towards evening. Despite this it is difficult to fall asleep - takes about 2 hours (I have not experienced sleep disturbance otherwise for some years). (14f10P)

Extreme exhaustion

Exhaustion, especially from late afternoon until evening. (2f/13)
All of a sudden very tired and grumpy in the afternoon. Feel completely shattered and worn out, don't feel like doing anything, everything and everyone is getting on my nerves. (8f/3)
Totally exhausted in the afternoon. (15f/15)

Exhaustion alternating with increased productivity

Tending towards exhaustion alternating with productivity. (15f/P)

Not tired in the evening, can't sleep, nevertheless full of energy in the morning

Go to bed at 11.00 pm but am actually not tired. I toss and turn, and wake up repeatedly in the night; am very restless and at 6.00am already feel charged up with energy. (6m/1)

More active in the evening than usual

Tired - but have done a lot. Energy is very good again in the evening. (11f/6)
Tiredness during the day, more energy in the evening again. (11f/7)
More energy again in the evening. (11f/9)

Wide awake in the evening, thoughts flowing

Lie down to sleep in the evening, but then am wide awake (I really NEVER have problems getting to sleep). I lie in bed awake, then phone up a colleague, then still lying there awake I feel restless, agitated, thoughts coming into my head, not really understanding why. I fall asleep after midnight. (12m/2)

<u>Generally more energy than usual</u> [17]

Feel good and full of energy. (2f/6)
Feel good, am full of energy (2f/20)
Go to bed at 11.00 pm but am actually not tired. I toss and turn, and wake up repeatedly in the night; am very restless and at 6.00am already feel charged up with energy. (6m/1)
30% to 40% more energy. (11f/5)
I unfortunately no longer have the feeling of being charged with energy that I experienced during the proving. I would like to continue taking the remedy. (11f/P)
Overall, during this time, I have felt full of energy, very self confident, was in a good frame of mind, and I managed to get a lot done. (13m/P)
Mentally strong. (15f/4)

<u>Light and full of energy</u>

Continue to feel free and light, and full of energy. (11f/7)

---

17 On the other hand (see footnote 13) it is Farokh Master who lists Vitis (as the last of three rubrics) in WILL - strong will power (Synthesis).

Vitis vinifera proving

(Vitis viniferae cum fructibus – Red wine from the Ahrtal, Germany) [J. W]

Proving procedure & general conditions

The proving substance

I spent my childhood in a wine village in the Ahr valley (one of Europe's most northerly red wine areas). In this romantic red wine island in the north-west of Germany, which has buried itself away in the Vulkan Eifel landscape (between Bonn and Coblenz), wine has always had a very great commercial as well as a cultural significance. The winegrowers put in a tremendous amount of hard work throughout each year on the steep vine slopes of the Ahr in order to cultivate them, so that by the end of the year they will have produced a vintage of particularly high calibre.

The hard work in these vineyards can particularly be seen alongside the easygoing attitude and the revelling wine festivals - which likewise have been traditional in this region for a long time.

The largest area in this wine region has been planted with the Pinot Noir, the blue Spätburgunder. I chose this particular wine for my study. The remedy was made into a mother tincture from the ripe grape, some leaves and stems from the blue Spätburgunder ('Recher Herrenberg', 1997 vintage) from Christoph Bäcker's organic vineyard in Mayschoß.

The mother tincture was processed on the same day the grape was picked in 1997. Together with Ulrike Wölbert, my assistant at the time, a colleague and biologist Dr. Gisela Nordhorn-Richter and the pharmacist Sven Göbel, the original substance was triturated up to the 3c potency[18] in lactose and then potentised up to 200c in alcohol in the Löwen Apotheke in Meckenheim

Study methodology

The study commenced in November 1997 in Bonn and the surrounding area, with colleagues who were alternative practitioners and midwives, and who had been attending my homeopathy study group for some years.

12 provers took the remedy (11 women and 1 man). Each prover was allocated a supervisor, who observed and supported the prover during the time of the study (approximately 6 weeks). Neither provers nor supervisors had knowledge of the substance being proved. The remedy was only then disclosed following a very lively concluding discussion as a group and once all provings symptoms had abated. Each supervisor took the respective prover's case prior to the proving in order to be able to differentiate between new and old symptoms and susceptibilities. The provers were to record in their proving journals all physical, mental and emotional changes in themselves that either they noticed personally, or that were noticed by their supervisors or others.

New, unfamiliar and unusual symptoms were to be particularly highlighted in the proving journals. It was these symptoms alone that were considered during the extraction process and they have been included in the following proving text.

On the basis of the number of provers participating the pharmacist provided a coded range of various potencies in globules, so that I too wouldn't know which prover had been given which potency.

Vitis vinifera cum fructibus was proved in 200c by 2 provers, 30c by 7, and 3 were given placebo (however prover 4 quit for a short time which meant we were

---

18 § 270 Samuel Hahnemann, Organon of Medicine, 6th edition

left with only 2 placebo provers). In the many homeopathic provings that have been conducted in the recent years it has become evident that placebo provers likewise develop clear symptoms from the proving substance, as if they had actually taken the remedy. For this reason I decided to include those prominent and striking symptoms experienced by the provers on placebo (they are marked clearly) in order not to miss out on their equally valuable experiences.

The first dose was taken collectively on the same day and at the same time, on 11th November at 7.30 am. It was continued 3 times daily until the first sign of noticeable changes, for a maximum of 2 days.

The proving journals

The following study deals with the listing of the original proving symptoms. I have used thematic headings in the chapters to provide better access to the 'disturbance of the vital force', specific to Vitis. In front of each symptom is the provers number, followed by the potency, and then the day it first appeared and, when available, the time of day. The first day is 'O'. 11 is the only male prover.

Mind

Isolated - Apathetic - Indifferent- Subdued - Slowed down - Composed

1.30.1
Feeling cut off, from people and events around me and also from my own feelings. I am not really involved, nothing really gets through to me.
1.30.18
Feel floppy, subdued, apathetic. Feeling 'bored with life'. Nothing really affects me, feel neither joy nor sadness.
1.30.21
I am apathetic and subdued.
1.30.22
Distortion of perception, several times during the day, each time lasting half a minute: blurred vision, vertigo. The impression: people and things are moving slower, including myself.
1.30.22
I continue to be subdued, slightly depressed, I feel nothing (lasts for a week).
1.30.28
I have decided to discontinue the proving today as a result of my emotional state. From my experience of taking homeopathic remedies in the past I am aware that I react strongly to them. My impression has been that since the beginning of the proving the energy available for me has been steadily dipping. There was a constant increase in physical and psychological tiredness, which finally expressed itself in the last week in problems with my circulation and distortion in my perception, which is extremely unusual for me. I had the impression that this remedy disturbed my rhythm of life to a great degree. The time when I have most energy is generally the evening, and I was deprived of this by the early evening and often experienced sudden tiredness.
As this symptom disappeared immediately after drinking a coffee to discontinue the proving, it seems obvious that it could have only been attributed to the remedy.
10.30.1.6:40
I takes me a while to get going.
10.30.3.6:40
It's taking me a long time to wake up today.
I've got the impression it's taking me a long time getting things done this morning.
10.30.23.9:30
I look out of the window. It has been snowing. The house is quiet. I can hear an ambulance and the fire brigade outside. I also feel detached from the goings on in the world here as well. I even fall asleep for 20 minutes while sitting.
11.30.8
My supervisor phoned. She sounded in a bad mood, I couldn't care less.

10.30.0.14:15
I'm absolutely tired out again and have a lie down on the sofa, sleep soundly until 3.00 pm.
I am not really affected by what the children say, although I take note of it.
6.30.50
Regarding my work morale:
Not very conscientious, just do what is necessary, like to take it easy, almost too much. It doesn't bother me that I haven't even made a start on all the things I intended to do.

Sitting still - Pondering
10.30.3.11:30
Want to sit down, sit quietly and ponder.

Asceticism - Abhorrence
11.30.13
Aversion to cigarette smoke. I am frequently overcome with a peculiar feeling of abhorrence yet I experience pity when I see others smoking. It is really evident to me how addiction eats away at people. Probably a more intense feeling because I was once into asceticism.

Contact - Communication - Cheerful - Fun - Pleasure
2.200.10.50
Retrospective observation:
It was obvious that I was feeling a lot calmer and relaxed, and others could see it in me.
In the foreground there was mostly an increase in communication, feeling well adjusted and cheerfulness.
2.200.0.21:30
I am in a very cheerful frame of mind this evening. I am relaxed and communicative.
2.200.2.16:00
I feel well in general, open and communicative, calmer than usual.
2.200.5.7:00
Feel fit and full of energy, but also nervous.
Deal with the work waiting to be done in a hectic manner, a lot of inner restlessness.
2.200.8.13:00
Full of energy again at the dance course and am enjoying learning.
2.200.10.9.00
A lot of energy and in the mood for work despite feeling like I've got a cold.
11.30.4
Really can't be bothered with my supervisor, would like to have nothing to do with her and keep in touch only when I feel like it.
11.30.6
Don't feel like making contact at all. They are too boring for me (seminar participants).

3.30.4
Feel well-adjusted psychologically, but no pleasure in my Tao seminar, putting up resistance.
11.30.11
I am not very communicative when in contact with others. I am not into arguing. Yet I express my opinions firmly, in a gentle way.
10.30.0.12:30
Am completely calm, able to devote myself to my child (rehearsing for school).
10.30.0.16:15
I take everything with great ease. Not affected by other people's problems.
12.30.25
Final observation:
In my family and work life there is always a lot going on. Particularly before Christmas. On the one hand I enjoy all these activities, on the other I am overcome with a kind of anxiety that excessive demands will be put upon me. Anxiety that I won't get it all done, don't have things under control. Then I usually fall into a kind of depression, which is not visible to others.
This sequence of events did not take place this year and everything went well, thanks to the proving remedy! I took everything much calmer, things were flowing well. I was not so inhibited and insecure.

Clear - Focused - Decisive
5.200.37
I often think about taking the remedy again. It's by my bed and I often hold it in my hand because I think it'll help me.
I am becoming more decisive, I re-experience emotional connections from the past with great clarity, as if a curtain had been pulled aside. It is painful, but it moves into the distance, as if in a different life.
2.200.10.50
Retrospective observation:
It was obvious that I was feeling a lot calmer and relaxed, and others could see it in me.
In the foreground there was mostly an increase in communication, feeling well adjusted and cheerful.
6.30.50
All in all during the proving I was able to make many decisions with a clear head. I purchased a new car, have created better boundaries for myself in the family. I was so clear about my decisions that no-one could doubt them.
12.30.0.12:00
Concentration is better. Better at reading a book, without falling asleep.
12.30.3.11:00
Considerably easier to do day-to-day things than before the proving. I feel resilient and composed.
10.30.15
I feel very efficient.

2.200.10.18:00

What astonishes me is that I feel full of energy despite feeling like I've got a cold. Can work and am very focused.

<u>Confusion - Difficulty concentrating - Beside myself - Mistakes - Fog - Trance - Stupid in the head</u>

1.30.1

My knees feel like they don't belong to my body, a little like they had been pumped up, not painful.

1.30.21

While walking I suddenly got an optical impression that the ground beneath me was swaying and caving in, > sitting.

2.200.8.13:00

Not able to concentrate at work and exhausted.

I feel very tired at midday, also still exhausted after an afternoon nap.

2.200.9.10:00

I slept for a long time, but feel very exhausted, not capable of concentrating on my work. I would prefer not to have to do anything at all and flap (like a chicken) between the kitchen and the office without accomplishing much.

Strong feelings of grief again, the first time since taking the remedy, feels more like a paralysis of energy.

6.30.Day 7,8,&9!

I am too confused to write anything down.

6.30.11

I can think and write again in an organised manner today, the confusion has subsided.

8.Plac.0.12:45

Somehow I don't feel in my body today. In the shop I had the feeling I was going through the motions of shopping but wasn't really there.

9.Plac.0.8:05

Feeling as if I was wrapped up in cotton wool (as if I'd taken valium).

9.Plac.0.9:55

Feeling as if someone else was fastening my shoelaces.

9.Plac.4.12:20

I want to phone my brother, dial a number. As the phone rings at the other end I realise that I have dialled the wrong number. I think about which number I dialled and realise that I dialled a number that has not existed for two and a half years.

9.Plac.29

Since the proving I am aware that I am getting words mixed up frequently or mix up the first letters of two words.

10.30.0.10:40

Drag myself around the flat, tired and floppy.

Difficulty reading, head is muzzy, almost as if in a trance.
And what do I do with the morning now?
Read pharmaceutical publicity and don't understand what has been written.
11.30.4.
I am driving to a seminar. During the journey I begin to doubt whether I am going to the right town. I look for the directions; I have left everything at home.
12.30.0.10:00
Try to read a book. But I keep falling asleep all the time. On one occasion I wake up with such a terrible shock, that a violent jerk goes right through me
10.30.0.11:10
Can't find my journal. I am not usually so forgetful. Could I have lost it?
10.30.2.21:00
Can't keep my eyes open when reading at my desk. I don't understand what I have just read.
10.30.10.17:30
Feel stupid, can't find the book I am looking for.

Absent-minded
5.200.0
I'm a bit absent-minded, but composed when working.
5.200.4
Have slight nausea, doubt myself and feel tired and exhausted.
Am very absent-minded.

Flapping like a chicken
2.200.9.10:00
I slept for a long time, but feel very exhausted, not capable of concentrating on my work. I would prefer not to have to do anything at all and flap (like a chicken) between the kitchen and the office without accomplishing much.
Strong feelings of grief again, the first time since taking the remedy, feels more like an immobilization of energy.

Time (mistakes in) - Appointments - Young - Old - Beautiful
2.200.9.17:00
Feeling exhausted before and after midday nap. I am shocked that the day is almost over.
3.30./
Feel stressed, everything is too much, not enough quiet time, too many leisure activities.
3.30.25
Lacking concentration very much when driving the car in the morning. The feeling of dashing through the days that I have had over the last weeks is very noticeable - too many things, people and appointments placing demands on me.

56

As I get home around 1.00 pm I notice there are a lot of dishes from the previous evening that need washing up. A friend is due to come round for a coffee at about 4.00 pm and then the family to celebrate Christmas Eve at around 8.00 pm. While I'm washing the dishes I'm realising that it's probably not going to work out time-wise. I can accept the fact that I will actually have to be talking to someone soon, but feel completely swamped and in some sense have lost the plot. As my friend arrives I am actually not in a position to chat to him. I am not able to think. I need a long time to understand a simple question and am only concerned with what is going on for me. It makes me feel anxious. I don't want to see anyone. He leaves worried and I tell him I have had too much going on recently and this is the result of it all.

After he has left I lie down in bed even though I am not tired. It's all too much for me, I need somewhere to shelter. The thought of visitors puts me in such an immediate panic that I contact my parents and cancel.

I feel the immense pressure growing in me when I am on the phone, and start to cry. I cry throughout the whole conversation, explaining it's just all too much for me, and that I would prefer not to see anyone. I already fell better for crying.

After the phone call I lie on the bed in the dark and the panic circles in my head, the feeling of cracking up, not being able to cope with anything else, everything is too much. I want to escape from every stimulus, every demand and I wonder how I am going to carry on. At the same time my rational side deliberates whether 'this is a nervous breakdown, what can you do to switch off, you will have to have peace and quiet'.

In the end a thought comes into the panic that it's my own fault if I lose the plot because I suppressed my athletes foot, instead of putting up with the symptoms. And then suddenly I had a thought that this could be to do with the proving. The thought alone shatters the panic cycle (I wondered briefly whether I could have taken cannabis or other drugs by mistake, as once, after unwittingly consuming 2 pieces of hash cake, it was impossible to concentrate and I felt that my ability to think were falling to pieces). I suck a Fisherman's friend (in an attempt to antidote) and try to get in touch with my supervisor in desperation. 15 minutes later I feel considerably better, and also notice that I have abdominal pains and am sufficiently back to my old self, that I am able to get myself to the bath. The attack is finally over after approximately 90 minutes. I feel completely exhausted, but once again 'feel the ground under my feet', can think clearly and the panic has gone.

I have never before experienced such a crisis as today, not even in times of extreme stress and at present I am neither under pressure in my private life, nor my work life. After this night I still feel somewhat distressed and can't integrate what I have experienced. Am I going round the bend or is this a symptom from the proving?

It has distressed me how close sanity and insanity are to each other.

Looking back on the last weeks I feel I have been agitated much more often and have taken on too much.

5.200.17

A lot of people have said I look younger. Things are not affecting me as much at the moment, more

able to distance myself from things.
6.30.3
A very stressful day, I had lots of appointments. I am irritable, no patience with children.
6.30.50
My sense of time is all mixed up, I am late with everything I've arranged. It keeps coming to me as a shock how time is flying by.
10.30.9:20
For the first time ever we get to the nursery so late that we have to ring the door bell.
10.30.0.9:55
Feel I didn't put the same vigour in getting the housework done as usual, but get it done in time.
10.30.0.10:00
I don't quite know what to do with my time at the moment.
10.30.0.11:10
I am sitting on the sofa and looking at the colourful red cherry tree and let time pass by (idly). Feel somehow detached from the dimension of 'time'.
10.30.2.18:00
Having difficulty with time. Half an hour seems like 10 minutes.
10.30.2.21:00
I keep looking at the calendar because I have noticed that I am having difficulty with time and appointments. I don't want to forget or miss out on anything.
10.30.3.7:00
I am a day ahead of myself. I put pressure on my son to get up even though he's not in school early until tomorrow.
10.30.3.7:50
I have been having thoughts of a philosophical nature:
>   *- What does the 'I' in people amount to?*
>   *- To what extent does habit affect people?*
>   *- To what extent can a proving remedy disrupt the normal (almost healthy) balance of a person?*
>   *- Do we first notice the effect in the difference of the rhythm?*
>   *- Can people who don't have a steady rhythm of life prove remedies at all?*
I feel a heaviness that makes me sit down and reflect.
10.30.3.8:00
I experience a disassociation with time.
10.30.3.13.30
I read an article in the 'Zeit' magazine. I was particularly interested in the article: Ask Dr. Proust, or In Search of Lost Time (Novel by Marcel Proust).
10.30.4.20.15
I watched the adventure of Odysseus on the television and saw parallels with the proving:
- Odysseus thought he had been there 5 days, but it was 5 years.

58

- *Odysseus was the first person to use his intellect and to act accordingly. He had to constantly be thinking and acting in different ways (to gouge out the Cyclops' eye).*
10.30.23.18:30
Feel old and stiff.
10.30.23.19:00
Today is the darkest day of the proving. I am thinking a lot and establish that the themes I have been dreaming about are my themes and not those of the proving remedy. 'Mid-life crisis'!!! For the first time I review the proving, and everything is clear to me.
10.30.25
Final observation:
I look back at a time when I felt how it was to be 'detached' from time (in a completely positive way). There was none of the typical pre-christmas stress for me leading up to christmas. I was able to organise my time. All the hustle and bustle drifted past me. I was able to perceive it in others, but didn't get swept away myself. I was completely calm and was able to draw up a solid plan for my days and weeks ahead, test it out and found it worked well for me.
It was very noticeable that once the proving symptoms subsided things fell back into the 'old ways'.
11.30.5
I am sitting in a seminar and thinking about how much homeopathy changes people. It makes them beautiful - in a unique way - and young.

<u>Depression – Self doubt - Subdued - Meaning</u>
3.30.8
A subdued feeling after a crucial conversation with a woman who has just given birth. Self doubt.
3.30.9
Subdued mood, worried, am annoyed by trivial things.
3.30.11
Very depressed on waking, everything looks grey, negative thoughts about work. No interest in anything, everything is too much. My mood improves as the day progresses, > in company. My mood improves once I take more interest in myself, put on make-up and wear bright colours.
3.30.15
Very bad mood, depressed leading to despair and aggression. Lack of concentration, self doubt, no reason behind it (11.00 am until the evening).
Mood is better after having a bath.
Very impatient and aggressive after being woken in the night.
3.30.19
Subdued mood, flat feeling, > after a walk in the fresh air.
10.30.23
When I asked my son if I can help him because he's got so much to do he tells me I should do something 'worthwhile'. I am very offended. I give what he said a lot of thought and have probably taken it too much to heart.

I have the feeling that I am being torn away from work (doing something useful) as soon as I begin anything.
10.30.23
I am almost depressed, everything seems so difficult. Feelings of heaviness (keep crying while making pizza).

<u>Aggressive - Irritable</u>
3.30.15
Very bad mood, depressed leading to despair and aggression. Lack of concentration, self doubt, no reason behind it (11.00 am until the evening).
Mood is better after having a bath.
Very impatient and aggressive after being woken in the night.
9.Plac.0.10.05
My car won't start (I left the lights on). I am fed up as I don't like driving our van. The thermos flask has fallen over, and is broken.
9.Plac.3.16:30
During an argument with my son I become so furious and start to scream that I am shocked by my behaviour.
11.30.15
Throughout the day irritable more frequently, and quicker than usual.
11.30.15
Quick to anger because my wife arrives an hour late for an engagement.
I confront her straight away and become immediately furious. My feeling is not to rely on others, particularly when they arrive late.

<u>Inner peace - Harmony</u>
2.200.7.7:00
Once again a surprising amount of energy, warmth and inner peace.
3.30.1
Considering my stressful work situation I am very well-balanced.

<u>Tough exterior</u>
6.30.6.15:00
I went to see '7 Years in Tibet' at the cinema. I am deeply impressed with how Peter Harrer [19] *loses his tough exterior.*

---

19 The explorer portrayed in this film is actually called Heinrich Harrer - and his colleague is Peter Aufschnaiter: could this be confusion, mistake or mix up related to Vitis or just a accidental mistake when recording the symptom?

<u>Sensitive - Tearful</u>
6.30.50
I am noticeably more sensitive. Cry very easily when people ask me about things that bother me. I am also not so affected by the suffering of others, that I would let myself be taken advantage of - or put myself second.
12.30.4.19:00
I read my daughter the fairy tale 'The little match girl'. I was so overwhelmed by the sadness in the story, that I could only carry on reading in fits and starts.

<u>Cleaning obsession</u>
10.30.0.9:55
A thought races through my head. Could I be obsessed with cleaning? I want everywhere to be clean, notice every bit of dust on the floor.

<u>See-saw process</u>
10.30.24
It becomes clear to me that I am going through some kind of see-saw process at the moment, also sexually, sometimes strong desire and sometimes none at all.

<u>Wanting to take the remedy</u>
5.200.66
I keep wanting to take the remedy

Dreams

Prover 10, who is a very reliable prover, experienced particularly intense dreams (before this proving she would only be aware of dreams on rare occasions). She also had a very strong reaction to the remedy in other ways. I have listed her 'flood of dreams' according to themes at the end of this chapter and kept them separate from the other provers' dreams.

<u>Cutting the face off - Severing the head - Mutilation - Death, child mutilation - Killing - No face</u>
2.200.10   Dream
I have cut off my husband's face with a bread knife, from the hairline to the chin. I feel very detached, more like a doctor operating. I feel neither aggression nor sympathy. More like a feeling of this is what needs to be done.
I am very careful not to cut the carotid artery. That would kill him. In the end I've got the whole

face in my hand, it is still connected to the neck and I don't know how to go on. No feelings attached to this, more like an astonishment.
Then I wake up.

12.30.12
I wake after a short dream.
It has to do with dead people. Someone has been decapitated with a knife.

3.30.7   Dream
I was at a film preview at the cinema in which an plane crashes (the film is called 'Mystery'). It explodes in the air and the middle part is spinning fast around it's own axle. After the crash I notice there is dead man who is half in, half out. A young boy who has survived is crawling behind him; he only has the part of his trunk containing his heart and lungs left, and a (left) stump up to the middle of his upper arm, everything else has been torn off. He's not bleeding. He is horrified as he begins to realise the extent to which he has been mutilated. Suddenly I am in the film and experience his horror. Then I wake up.

3.30.4   Dream
I visit a couple I have been looking after as a midwife and establish that the baby has died in the uterus.
It is a calm dream, no horror. (This actually happened to a colleague of mine 2 months ago).

5.200.2   Dream
I had a terrible nightmare during the night, someone was going to kill me. I was very tiny in the dream, a shudder went through my body.

11.30.7   Dream
I am standing in front of a villa - a strange building, old, yet a modern design, a lot of glass and high rooms, 3-4 storeys. It's a magnificent house. It belongs to my aunt and uncle. They want to hand it down to us, but on the condition that we live there as well. I am without any doubt that I could only move in if neither of them were living in the house with us. My wife and daughter go for a walk - the villa is on the edge of a forest. I am standing on the street, a car drives past. I suspect foul play. A man and a woman get out of the car, they have no faces. Dogs get out of the car with them as well. Alsatians. Only one of them poses a threat to me - the largest one. It takes a bite at my right arm, I can't fend him off. My arm disappears into his maw, up to my elbow. I am okay. At the same time there's a group of children, about 6-10 years old. They want to take something from me, I don't know what it is. They pounce on me and want a fight with me. I have to shake them off. They pinch, kick and hit me. I find it necessary to have to hit them back, as I don't know how else to defend myself. It depresses and torments me.

Car - Blood test - To be a man or a woman - Female friend - Dying the hair
9.Plac.3   Dream
When visiting a female friend I dyed my hair black.

7.30.0.7:30   Dream
The dream takes place in England. I have parked my car there somewhere. Then the car has disappeared and there is a building site where the car park used to be. People know where the car is, but I have to have a blood test. The blood test is to find out whether I am a man or a woman. Then I don't get my car back (I am distraught).

9.Plac.3   Dream
When visiting a female friend I dyed my hair black.

9.Plac.8   Dream
I am in the sauna with my husband and female friend. But I only want to go into the steam room with my female friend. As soon as my husband comes in I leave.

Marriage - Theatre
9.Plac.2   Dream
I am marrying my husband for a second time. But when I'm in the church I ask myself whether it's such a good idea to marry him. Friends of ours had already been up to the altar. They were sitting opposite each other on stools. Do they want to present something? They would have to get up again though, as a 35 year old woman was being baptised.

Cheating - Discipline - Cigarettes - Lift
2.200.11.   Dream
My daughter and I are sitting at the table, we're trying to work something out. We've got a card with 6 boxes printed on it, and we have to put girls names in the boxes and then assign the names to those of birds. What makes this complicated is that we are supposed to know the girls, but not know them well. This is difficult and we cheat a bit ie we also put names of well-known girls down. Then I wake up. I am surprised about the cheating, as I would normally not cheat in the presence of my daughter.

12.200.14.   Dream
Sitting in a hotel room with Anne and a female colleague, we are working.
The hotel is enormous, lots of floors. We are on somewhere around the 18th floor. I want to go down and get some cigarettes. That's going to take me ages. The colleague asks me to bring her some herbs from my room.
Reception is right at the bottom, where is my room?? Higher up in the building via long corridors and a lift.

63

This is going to take a while. I think Anne is going to be fed up if I leave the group for such a long time and won't want to work with me afterwards. But then I decide to go anyway.

First of all I take the lift to reception. I get confused on the way and am not sure which floor my room is on - because of the herbs. I think that if I go down first of all, I'll then know where to go. Then I wake up.

Gold
5.200.13
Dreams of gold (unfortunately no further recollection of this dream).

Tom-cat has a fall - Accidents
5.200.65
After dreaming that my tom-cat had a fall (belly flop) I fall when coming out of a friend's front door. I've grazed and bruised myself and I'm in a lot of pain. My purse has fallen under a car. I pick up all my things and spend the whole evening lying on the sofa with my cat. My thoughts about this: I am getting old. I was talking about the Fountain of Youth and themes to do with addiction today. I will have to keep moving otherwise I will cease up.

Building a house - Neighbour's garden - View
8.Plac.2.   Dream
We want to build a house. In doing this we would, however, spoil the view, or rather block the neighbour's view. And so we decide against it.

Reading at mass
12.30.25   Dream
I am supposed to do a reading at mass. Despite a mad rush I arrived a few minutes late. When it was time for me to recite the lesson I could only do so with great difficulty. It was not written at all clearly. Also it was very dark, and there was only dim lighting in the room.

Tree on the hillside - Powerful horse
11.30.14   Dream
I want to go to a homeopathy seminar. I don't know where it is and who's organising it. It makes me feel sad, because I don't want to go to that place. I am standing under a tree on the grass with two other people. The tree is on the hillside. A beautiful, powerful horse gallops up the hillside and gets down on its knees behind me. I sit in front of it and lean my back against the horse. It protects and comforts me.

Prover 10's dream journal

<u>Journey - France - Old ruins - Unruly child on the scaffolding - Fall from the 3rd floor to the ground</u>
10.30.0.6:00   Dream

I fall asleep again after the alarm has gone off and then have a nightmare: We are in France, living in a rather old-fashioned place that is falling apart and I am in charge of the catering. For the journey home I take what's left of the provisions. Then we go back into the town one more time. All of a sudden my son has disappeared. I find him scrambling around on the scaffolding, without any inhibition. He jumps from the 2nd floor and lands jubilantly on his feet. It is time for us to be making a move for our journey home. We'll make our way back. M. also comes. I make friends with a French woman - she tells me all sorts of things on the way home. But now I have to interrupt her suddenly because I have seen St. - the little rascal - climbing back on the scaffolding. I run after him calling him, and leave the French woman behind. I carry on shouting, louder and louder, that he shouldn't be messing around on the scaffolding. But then he runs even quicker along the planks and falls off the 3rd floor of the scaffolding, head first. I wake up as he hits the ground. Thank god it's only a dream!!!

I'm thinking about things longer than I usually do this morning; I never have dreams like this usually! Then I have to get a move on in the bathroom, even here things aren't working out like they usually do.

<u>Indoor swimming pool, lake - Green bathing costume - Cloakroom key - Clothes disappear - No panic</u>
10.30.1.   Dream

We had gone for a swim together (my husband and I). It was somewhere in an indoor swimming pool quite a distance away, but before then, in a lake. I swam the whole of the time, on my back. It was unbelievably beautiful. I was wearing a green swimming costume. There were colleagues from the past there, but we didn't speak to each other or make contact. When it was time to go home I couldn't find the key for the cloakroom. And the locker that I put my clothes in is empty. I'm not panicking at all, trusting that if I look for long enough then I'll find everything. Somebody says that the clothes were in the train, which had already left and they'd be on it when it returned. I look in the cubicles and lockers and realise that there's nothing here on wheels. Then I wake, hesitantly. I actually want to carry on looking for them. It takes a while before I come out of the dream into the real world.

<u>Spain, on holiday - Quaint wooden wall panelling - Greedy fish - Cloudy water - Caretaker - Toilets - Tram - Track - Bridging with a piece of wood</u>
10.30.2.   Dream

We're on holiday (Spain). We're doing a lot of sight-seeing. We're in a large Natural History Museum. Very old fashioned, with lots of quaint wooden wall panelling. Amongst other things there are some greedy fish in a pond. They can be fed through a special device so that people can see their teeth. The aquarium is full of fish food. I think that the poor fish will be completely overfed, and the water has already turned cloudy and stinks. There is a lot of commotion in this part of the museum.

There's a dangerous situation: One of the visitors is a threat to the museum caretaker. The caretaker is, however, unaware of the danger. We want to help - it has something do with hiding a pole, approximately one meter in length. I am not sure whether the caretaker and this peculiar visitor are in cahoots.

I am able to throw the pole down to a landing on the stairs. The exit from the museum is through the toilets. I go there a lot, on one occasion I can't shut the doors, but this doesn't bother me. We decide to go back by tram as only some members of the family had finished looking round. The tram comes every hour at 7 minutes past the hour and leaves at 10 past. We think about whether to take the earlier one (just after 6.00 pm) or the later one. We see the tram arriving and leaving. A piece of the track is missing and has been bridged with a piece of wood.

Supervisor's TV - Old contraption
10.30.2   Dream (2)

My supervisor gives me a television. An old contraption (possibly black and white) but in good working order.

Preparations for a party - Defrosting chicken - Unfriendly
10.30.3.   Dream

I have to prepare the food for a party for a lot of people. I go to the butcher's as early as 5 days before to find out how long chicken takes to defrost. The staff are very unfriendly, as they're very busy. They are more interested in selling than giving advice. A female shop assistant says very impolitely: 'You will just have to get up at 3.00am and defrost them, that's what we have to do'. I feel quite offended. The slogan being: Excuse me, but you should be allowed to ask for advice when you have to plan things in advance.

Choosing furniture - But not wanting to buy - Noticed - Annoyed
10.30.4.   Dream

We're looking at furniture. We listen to the advice given, but actually already know that we don't want to buy anything from them, as we intend to go somewhere else. At some point they notice this in the furniture shop and are annoyed with us.

Friend – Bike tour - Domestic obligations - Hats - Moving from ground floor to 5th floor - Old piano - Up the stairs - Down the stairs - Art nouveau, dark wood
10.30.6   Dream

I am supposed to be spending some time with a male friend. We were supposed to be going on a bike tour and going for a swim. I told him I can't because I'm busy. I have to take care of my household chores, shopping, cleaning and to help my mother move. She has a hat shop and is moving it from the ground floor to the 5th floor. Piles of hats have to be carried up the stairs, as well as carpets, which also have to be washed. I live where my parents' old shop used to be, in the attic. My friends are annoyed about my domestic obligations and insinuate that I have overestimated the time I need for the cleaning, and that it is not such a large area. I argue that there is also the washing to do and that I have so much tidying up to do beforehand. In addition I also need to help with the move.

When we come to have a break from carting the hats around and have something to eat (midday) I notice an old piano and I can't hold back from playing a few notes on it. It 's almost like an organ, above the keyboard there is another enclosed keyboard which can be opened to access the lower notes. The landlord comes and says I have to stop playing, and should carry on with helping with the move. But this is break time, and I am somewhat peeved. Then we carry on with the move, carting things up and down the stairs. To get back down I have developed a fantastic technique for jumping down and we also optimize on carrying the hats.

There are old, art nouveau style iron windows with folding shutters in a dark wood, and generally there's a lot of dark wood. The room is a triangular shape, how will we get all the hats to fit in. I don't think it's such a good idea anyway, having a hat shop so high up in a building. How are the customers (older women) to be expected to get up to the top when there's no lift. Suddenly I'm getting a bit concerned about the pile of hats, whether some of them might have dents in them.

Mind mapping - Theatre square
10.30.6   Dream

I wanted to take part in a seminar on mind-mapping. I have already received information about it through the post, and lots of forms that can be sent in if you want advice and feedback. Some time later (I didn't get round to filling in the paperwork and sending it off) I heard that a lot of people attended the seminar (600 participants). I felt sad that I didn't get round to filling in the forms and post them. Then there's a complete change of scenery and I am walking in my home town through Theatre Square.

Journey in the van - Farmer - Washing lines - Washing lines up to the trees - Sodden mountain meadow - Mountain slope - Dismantled wheels - Roots, tree stump - Down the slope
10.30.7   Dream

I am in our van, driving to our farmer's. I always buy fruit and vegetables there. I can also have a nice chat to the farmer's wife about lots of things, including things to do with the home and things like that. Today we're talking about the washing. She tells me that she has already hung up her five children's trousers on the line (4 or 5 full machine loads). As I'd like to stay there longer I hang my washing up as well, on washing lines that go from the bus up to the trees (as when camping).

Change in scenery: Our van is on the hillside on rather sodden ground. The farmer owns the land. The path leading to the meadow is pretty boggy. Where our van has been parked, the ground had been levelled with large rocks so that the van can stay upright. When we come to drive away we notice that our front wheels have been dismantled and the suspension had been damaged. My husband steps into action and gets the farmer's son to help him. I start to become concerned about whether we can get down to the bottom of the hillside in the van in one piece. In the meantime it starts to sleet and we women have to take the washing in so it doesn't get wet again. We manage to get this done. On the way down there are some roots and a thick tree stump right on top. The only way to get past would be in a jeep. There are however a variety of small cars driving down the hillside and when they come to this point they just drive alongside the track. I'm just concerned about the width of our van, but my husband says it'll work out fine.

Open day - Painting a friend's body - Horse on a naked body
10.30.8   Dream

We're sitting in a lecture hall. A variety of subjects are covered, similar to an open day - each teacher talking about a topic. I'm full of enthusiasm. Then it's time for us to draw something. All of a sudden I'm doing a painting on a friend's body. She wants to have a large A and a horse painted on her naked body. You can see she's enjoying having it done. Her husband keeps popping his head around the door to see how I'm getting on.

Tidiness - Cleaning up - Shared house
10.30.8   Fragment of a dream

At my grandmother's house. Something to do with tidying up. Hoovering under mattresses. I am sleeping on an old sofa-bed that belongs to my grandmother, in the living room. It is very untidy. A group of people, as if it was a shared house.

Journey - Sliding into a hole leading into a cellar
10.30.9   Dream

Three of us have gone to a study group. As we're driving home we skid into a hole leading into a cellar. The body work under the car has broken into pieces. I suggest we could stick it together provisionally. There is doubt as to whether it will hold.

First communion - Summer festival - Beer at the hairdressers
10.30.10   Dream

People are celebrating first communion in my village. We are having a stroll through the village. The strange thing is that wherever you look people are having a good time, as if they were at a summer festival where there's a beer garden. We have a beer at the hairdressers even though we don't really want to have anything to do with all the fuss over the communion.

Trip in the van - Level-crossing - Overtaken
10.30.10   Dream

We are on our return journey from somewhere or other in our van: we take a left turning in Bach Street, so we can get across the level-crossing. But it's closed and we have to wait. We park the van appropriately and wait. But then suddenly we are overtaken by trucks and cars. They turn left just before the crossing and drive alongside across the tracks. More and more cars keep doing this. I'm beginning to get concerned about what'll happen when the train comes!! What one earth are they doing there and why are they doing it!!??

Family holiday - Inclining conveyor belt - Fastening shoes together - Engine power - Weight on the shoulders, like a tug-of-war - Revolving door - Three-metre board, not for me

10.30.12   Dream

We are on holiday as a family, also with some friends and children. We are on bikes on the way to a farm. People can sleep in the hay on the farm. Everyone had to bring a sleeping bag. There is also a swimming pool. The shoes and sleeping bags had to be put on a kind of conveyor belt. When they come to the end the shoes are then tied together into pairs by some kind of automatic mechanical action, and the sleeping bags are folded up or rolled up. I am interested in how the machine works and find out that a great deal of power is needed for the drive propulsion system. The conveyor belts (at least four of them) are in a large, rectangular pit and incline at the end. I am allowed to help a man with one of the belts. We have to pull really hard on an iron chain. It is over his shoulder, goes forwards and I get hold of the end of it, which is hanging down to the ground in front of him. It is similar to a tug-of-war. I pull on it with all my strength, walking backwards. I give it all I've got. But there's not enough momentum. The sleeping bag falls off the end of the conveyor belt again, unfolded. I don't understand it, he manages to do it on his own, how is that possible? The strange thing about this holiday accommodation is the revolving doors (similar to the ones in Cologne cathedral, only glass outside all around). We have to keep going through revolving doors. The entrance to the main building has doors like this, the swimming pool too. We even have to go through there with the bicycles. I am always a bit anxious when we have to go through these revolving doors. Looking at them from above they remind me of a wheel on my bicycle, the sections that separate the compartments are like spokes. At the end of the holiday, when it's time to go back home again, we have to round up the children (who had a great time there) as well as the bicycles and take them through these revolving doors again. While doing this, on the stairs I pass the window or exit where the three-metre board is, in the swimming pool. I take a peep and decide that I wouldn't like to dive from there. When only the bicycles remain to be taken through the revolving door it has suddenly changed. It is now wider and between 20 - 50 cm of it is in the open air. In addition to this there is a corridor alongside it, leading outside, which is curved, everything made of glass and there's another small revolving door. We are still waiting there for somebody and something. Teenagers are spinning the door round really fast. There's no need for me to be worried about any of then getting stuck as there's plenty of room for them. I nevertheless think it's dangerous.

Bus journey - Dealing with everything - Friendliness
10.30.13   Dream

I was travelling again, holiday, expedition. Exploring a foreign country, travelling on a public coach, coping with dangerous situations. People were very friendly to us wherever we went.

Teacher-centred learning - Cough - Mess - Music is explained - Mistakes are okay - Tinsel angel - Asian people in long habits
10.30.14.   Dream

I am at university. We are sitting in class being taught, I thinks it's maths. All of a sudden I have to cough. I want to get a lozenge out of my bag. My bag is a complete mess, lots of pens, and sweets, and everything falls out of my bag which disrupts the class quite a bit. There's a splashing sound coming from the benches behind me as if someone is having a pee. Then it's break time. I stroll with the others through the university building and peep into the lecture halls that are empty. I go into one of them where music is being taught. A piece of music is played in sections on a kind of organ and then explained. A very different lecturing method. People can come and go in the lecture hall. I like this kind of teaching. I see an old classmate from school in another row. I want to meet up with her later for a chat. At the end of the lecture students can volunteer to play the organ, and also excerpts from the music covered beforehand. People can have a go, and it's okay to make mistakes. This horrifies one female student who turns into a tinsel angel, hanging on the wall. The lecturer is applauded for her lecture and is presented with lots of flowers afterwards. She stuffs them rather disrespectfully into a large saucepan. Then everyone leaves. I carry on strolling through the university and wait for my old classmate. But she is nowhere to be seen. All of a sudden I am in flat similar to a castle. The whole place is full of old furniture; unoccupied by the looks of things. I take a look at everything. When I'm ready to leave I can't find the exit. Eventually I pick up the courage to ask a couple of people that I meet in one of the large rooms. They are young people, sitting on the floor. Then I find my way out straight away. Outside in the corridors it's like being on top of a large castle with cannon muzzles in the courtyard. I always wanted to go inside but it was always closed to the public. I take a close look at everything. At all the cannons in the courtyard. Then I leave the building and am back in the university turmoil once more.

Running with ease - Stout man - Swimming in a lake in the woods - Taking care of a child - Proud of myself
10.30.18   Dream

I'm on holiday. At some point I'm jogging across a field. An older, stout man joins me. I'm pleased how little effort I require to run, it's an amazing feeling in my body. It's pretty cold outdoors, we want to go for a swim after in a lake in the woods. We are then quite wet (our clothes) and need to change so we don't catch a chill. Then suddenly I have to take attend to one of my young children, it's priority. I'm trembling all over from being in wet clothes. It takes quite a long time and I notice how I'm getting warmer and warmer. The clothes have dried on me.
A wonderful feeling. I am somehow proud of myself how I'm coping with everything.

A boy has got Aids
10.30.18   Fragments of a dream

It is about a group of people (nursery school) and a boy has Aids. The question is how are we going to go about it.

Paris – All inclusive - Car disappears - Friendly people - Ticket inspection - Steps that are double the usual height - Chaos - Carrying my son
10.30.20   Dream

I am in Paris (with my husband, a child and a group of friends). We have booked a holiday with hotel, underground, tickets ...... all inclusive and also time to spend as we wish. We have a car of our own, bright yellow. We drive through the middle of Paris, find somewhere to park and go sightseeing. Then my husband wants to go back to the hotel, but I want to carry on sightseeing. So we split up. My son stays with me. We look at lots of things until we're tired. We just about manage to get back to the car park. But the car isn't there, my husband most probably took it back to the hotel. We go to the underground, where friendly people help us to find what we need and explain about the tickets. Tickets are being inspected on the underground. I've lost my ticket, I look in all my coat and trouser pockets and handbag. But I can't find the (pale yellow) ticket. The ticket inspector carries on. A second ticket inspector comes, I am completely at the end of my tether, but I only need to pay 20 cents as we are just about to pass the zone that the ticket would have been valid in. Then I can get the inspector to stamp a new ticket. I still had some new ones in my bag. People are amazingly friendly to me.

As we were making our way to our hotel, diagonally from the lower right hand side of the city map to the upper left, we found out that my husband and a colleague, who knows Paris well, had taken the car back. I notice houses with steps twice as high as they usually are. I have to carry my son, my bags; it's all pretty chaotic for me, and everything's got mixed up in my handbag. But the French are friendly (I wake feeling that the dream is not complete and want to carry on dreaming).

Workshop - Visit sister briefly - Wedding dress - Unreliability - Detached
10.30.22 Dream

We want to drive to a workshop, meet someone halfway and then take this person's car for the rest of the journey. I'll also be able to visit my sister there, just want to pop in, but then we start chatting. We start to feel tired and have a lie down (my sister, her husband and I in their bed, properly dressed in our pyjamas). After a while my sister gets up and decides to try her wedding dress on again. She maintains that she has put on weight over the last few years and wants to lose some. It occurs to me that what I actually wanted to do was to go to the workshop. I get dressed, it's all getting to be hectic. I want to put my trousers on over my pyjamas , but it's all bumpy. What on earth is going on, usually I am so reliable. Will they still be waiting for me outside? In addition, my sister's children are bothered by me getting dressed, because they want to sleep.

In all of these events I have the feeling that none of this has anything to do with me! I'm detached from it all!

<u>Trituration and proving - Paediatrician, son who is ill - Heartless - Heart prevailing</u>
<u>over reason</u>
10.23.24   Dream
I dream about a study group in which there were non-medical practitioners and a paediatrician. We
were discussing trituration and provings. I put my hand up and I have something to say about it. I
noticed how my contribution was received favourably and with acknowledgement, even by the
paediatrician. Then we want to repertorise a case. It's a live case, the doctor's young son actually.
He is very ill and the doctor examines him with us all present. In my opinion he is doing this in a
very heartless fashion, not at all how you would treat your own son. The little boy is very ill, mucous
and pus are oozing out of his ears, his face is red, his mouth and throat have a white coating.
When he has finished we want to repertorise the case. I want to get on with it as well and focus on
the most important aspects. But my heart has got the better of me. I ask if it's alright for me to look
after the little boy and take him to bed. He needs to be cuddled and feel cared for sometimes. And of
course I am given permission. In that moment I realise that this is just right for me. I come to life,
as I carry him in my arm; am able to stroke him, take him to bed, put on a fresh nappy. Then I
notice his sore bottom and back, how awful, something should be done about it, where's there some
cream? I look for it and then the doctor's wife comes. I am happy to be able to hand over the little
boy. Now we can get on with repertorising. In fact I now have additional information that will be
very useful. (This was a wonderful dream)

Vertigo

<u>Staggering – slowed down</u>
1.30.21
Whilst walking I suddenly had the impression, both as a feeling and visually, that the ground was
swaying and giving way, > sitting.
1.30.22
Distorted perception repeatedly during the day, each time lasting half a minute, blurred vision,
vertigo, the impression that people and things were moving at a slower pace, myself included.

<u>Drank too much (alcohol)</u>
5.200.11
I have been waking between 1.30 and 2.30 am on a regular basis with problems in my head to do
with circulation, which frighten me. I get up out of bed, feel like I've drunk too much alcohol. Feel
dizzy, then I get back to bed again, calm myself down and am able to fall asleep again.

Standing in front of the wash-basin - Getting up from the chair
10.30.1.6:40
Mild vertigo and empty sensation in my abdomen when standing in front of the wash-basin.
11.30.7.10:00
Vertigo from my ears upwards (not in the whole of my head) after getting up from the chair.
Pressure in my left breast lasting approximately 10 seconds, it comes and goes. I am somewhat concerned. Nothing has an effect on it.

Head

Itching - Dandruff - Hair loss
10.30.3.7:00
My head is itching dreadfully. More dandruff than normal when combing my hair, also hair loss.
10.30.5.8:00
Intense itching over the whole head, not improved by scratching. Large flakes of dandruff and scabs. Better from a hot shower and brushing hair.
10.30.7.13:30
Dandruff, almost as large as rolled oats, flaking off when scratching my head.

Heat
10.30.23.17:00
Heat in my head, yet feeling cold in my body, feel slightly chilly.

Bunged up
11.30.12.7:45
I feel ill, bunged up around my forehead. Blow my nose but there's nothing there.

Headache

Pressure - Wandering - Stabbing
2.200.1.7:30
Pressure in my forehead on waking, the whole forehead initially, then felt more on the left side and later over the whole head.
2.200.1.7:30
The headache starts off in my forehead, then moves around in the front of my head, at times stronger on the right side, at other times in the forehead. Feel the pain 'deep in my head'.
2.200.1.9:30
Mild twinges in my lower abdomen (ovaries?), starting off mild, right sided, then very noticeable on

73

the left side, with stabbing pain in my right temple simultaneously, then wandering, stabbing pain in my forehead.

2.200.3.10:45

Headache, pressing in my left temple, intense and lasting a long time, with a dull sensation in my head, > lying on my left (painful) side.

2.200.4.12:30

Pressure in my left forehead.

2.200.5.14:00

Pressure in my left temple.

5.200.1

Mild headache which increases gradually, felt as a pressure behind the eyes.

6.30.11

Dull pressure in my head beneath the skull and in my forehead.

Am able to think and write in an orderly fashion again, the confusion has subsided.

8.Plac.0.17:00

Mild pressure in my head behind my forehead and eyes, comes and goes.

Also mild nausea. Feels like the nausea is connected to the metallic taste I am experiencing.

11.30.11.13:00

Ground to a halt by midday and need to have a lie down. Feels like the flu, with some pressure in my left ear.

Also pressure in my head (forehead and skull) and eyes, with drawing sensation in the upper left molars.

Fresh air

3.30.19

Walking in the fresh air improves my headache.

From neck to the back of the head

3.30.20

Headache on waking which lasts the whole day. It starts at the neck, extending to the back of the head and forehead, more right than left and < from standing up quick. It improves after the evening meal.

Eyes

Warm - Hot

2.200.0.10:00

Heat in the hands and tired eyes.

11.30.13.18:00

74

I am conscious of my eyes, they feel hot, but I don't have any fever. Feeling of tension in the bronchial tubes and lungs.
11.30.13.
Sensation of heat internally, particularly in the mouth and pharynx, urethra, stomach and eyes, with a desire for cold water.
But I only drink a little as my body often feels chilled and I would prefer not to have to go out before or after 11.00 am to 4.00 pm.

Sensation of a foreign object
11.30.9
During the afternoon I often had the feeling there was a hair in my eye. I check it out but can't find anything. It irritates a bit.
11.30.10
Several times throughout the day I felt as if there was a hair under my right eyelid, causing a red discolouration of the conjunctiva.
11.30.11.13:00
Ground to a halt by midday and need to have a lie down. Feels like the flu, with some pressure in my left ear.
Also pressure in my head (forehead and skull) and eyes, with drawing sensation in the upper left molars.
I have noticed that I have been sneezing over the last couple of days, at varying intervals and keep feeling the need to blow by nose but there's no discharge.
I also have a sensation of a hair or grain of sand under my right upper lid. Makes me think of hay fever symptoms.
12.30.11.9:00
Felt like I'd got a foreign object in my right eye on the way to a seminar. I check it out in the mirror but can't find anything.
12.30.12
The same feeling again in the morning, as if there's something in my eye, this time affecting the left eye.

Tired - Heavy
10.30.2.21:00
While sitting at my desk can't keep my eyes open when reading. I don't comprehend what I've just read.

Cramp - Irritation
9.Plac.3.7:20
I rub my eye in such a awkward fashion that I poke my eyeball, which has caused some irritation to the eye.

10.30.5.17:30
Cramp in left eye muscles when reading.

Vision

<u>Blurred - Veil - Fog</u>
1.30.19.17:00
Poor circulation: debility, shaky legs, mild nausea, blurred vision, < sitting.
1.30.22
Distortion of perception, several times during the day, each time lasting half a minute: blurred vision, vertigo. The impression: people and things are moving slower, including myself.
10.30.7.21:30
A veil in front of my eyes while reading, like fog.

<u>Darkness</u>
10.30.18.17:45
Almost caused an accident on the way home after going to the farmer's. It was dark and I didn't see a delivery van coming from the left side. Only just missed by the skin of my teeth. Where did it come from?
10.30.18.18:00
Difficulty seeing in the dark.

<u>Reading</u>
5.200.1
Don't see so well, can't recognise capital letters.
10.30.18.20:00
Difficulty deciphering the programme at a concert. What is wrong with my eyes?

Ears

<u>Dull - Pressure - Plane</u>
11.30.6
Mild pain in my left ear (acoustic meatus) together with a numb sensation. The same as in an plane or something similar. Try to clear my ears several times but it doesn't help. External pressure aggravates the pain. It's still with me as I fall asleep.
11.30.11.13:00
Ground to a halt by midday and need to have a lie down. Feels like the flu, with some pressure in

my left ear.
Also pressure in my head (forehead and skull) and eyes, with drawing sensation in the upper left molars.

Itching
10.30.5.8:00
Intense itching over the whole head, not improved by scratching. Large flakes of dandruff, and scabs. Better from a hot shower and brushing hair.
And itching inside left ear.
12.30.21
Intense itching in the ears suddenly in the evening.

Electricity
12.30.0.8:00
Sensation like electric shocks in right ear after the first dose of the remedy, a couple of times in a row.
One minute later I notice the same sensation in the upper abdomen, but somewhat weaker.

Whistling
9.Plac.8.9:20
Short, high pitched whistling in right ear.

Nose

Sneezing - Tingling
2.200.10.4:00
Woken up by the dog barking.
Feel like I'm getting a cold.
Sneeze 2-3 times, severe tingling, only in right nostril.
Clear nasal discharge in right and left nostril, right is less blocked. .
2.200.10.18.00
Severe bouts of sneezing time and again throughout the whole day, tingling in the nose to some extent, < right side but also on the left.
Clear nasal discharge, excoriated nostrils.
10.30.19.19:45
Seemingly never-ending sneezing fits, followed by a runny nose.

Obstructed - Swollen
3.30.2

Blocked nose on waking, some discharge, and a need to blow my nose often. The mucous is pale yellow, viscous and only a small amount.

Once I'm up I can breathe through my nose again, during breakfast I have to blow my nose frequently, but after that not so often.

The mucous membranes in my nose have been swollen all day, but breathing is only affected slightly. I am better in the fresh air than indoors.

3.30.3

Blocked right nostril on waking, left is unaffected. Not much nasal discharge, light yellow to clear mucous. Sneezed once.

11.30.12.7:45

I feel ill, bunged up around my forehead. Blow my nose but there's nothing there.

11.30.13

Blocked nose with no discharge. Left nostril feels very dry. Left upper molars are very painful, as with maxillary sinusitis. Feel like I've got flu, but no fever.

11.30.14

Woke at 4 am again. Difficult to get back to sleep again this time. On top of this my nose was completely blocked.

Yellow - Bloody

2.200.10.9.00

The nasal discharge is now quite pale yellow, and not so much of it. Sneezing now and then. Now I've got just slight tingling, firstly left nostril, then right.

6.30.1.7:00

Nasal discharge initially pale yellow with some blood, then clear with light blood. Yellow discharge from the inside corner of the eyes.

11.30.19

Nose and pharynx severely congested with phlegm overnight, and I had to blow out and spit up large amounts of yellow to clear phlegm.

Face

Itching - Excoriated - Burning - Rhagades - Dry - Herpes

1.30.16.20:30

Spontaneous, intense itching under the lower lip with slightly red skin discolouration in this area and a small bump which looks like a grain of barley. Itching lasts for about 15 minutes, scratching does not >. Afterwards I only notice this area when I touch it, when it burns, as if it's excoriated.

2.200.1.7:30

The cracks in the corner of the mouth are very painful.

2.200.2.7:00

The cracks in the corner of the mouth are very painful.
2.200.2.16:00
The crack in the corner of the mouth is very painful and has crusted over.
A lymph node under the left side of the chin is swollen and is very painful when pressure is applied.
2.200.4.7:00
Intense burning, crack on left hand corner of mouth which has grown to about 4 times the size it was in the beginning, and has developed a yellow brown crust.
2.200.4.9:00
The crack doesn't burn any more, but any movement causes pain, laughing etc.
2.200.10.18.00
Severe bouts of sneezing, time and again throughout the whole day, tingling in the nose to some extent, < right side but also on the left.
Clear nasal discharge, excoriated nostrils.
6.30.12
Very dry mouth and lips, they still feel dry after a bottle of mineral water.
6.30.13
Mouth and lips are permanently dry.
Herpes starting under the nose, feels sore.
6.30.24
Herpes came on during menses, mouth and lips continue to be very dry, drinking does not give any relief.
7.30.20
Very dry in the corner of my mouth.
7.30.34
Corner of the mouth very sore and dry.
9.Plac.20
Herpes came on extremely suddenly on the left side of the upper lip. Tension in the lip.

Young - Swollen - Dirty
5.200.17
A lot of people have said I look younger. Things are not affecting me as much at the moment, more able to distance myself from things.
10.30.3.7:00
I look in the mirror and see I'm puffed up, as if I hadn't slept enough or went to bed too late yesterday, but that's not the case.
10.30.8.9:30
Throughout the day I keep getting the feeling that I hadn't washed my face today.

Warm – Glowing
2.200.0.16:00

Warm hands and face.
2.200.0.19:00
Warm face.
2.200.1.14:00
Warm hands and face
2.200.2.16:00
Generally warmer than usual, most noticeable on hands and face.
2.200.10.18:00
Felt frozen until 5.00 pm. Now I am lovely and warm, especially my hands and face.
10.30.0.10:40
Feel like my cheeks are red and glowing.

Mouth

Dry - Raw - Excoriated - Blisters
6.30.12
Very dry mouth and lips, they still feel dry after a bottle of mineral water.
6.30.13
Mouth and lips are permanently dry.
7.30.13.18:30
Small strip between lower jaw and lip is excoriated, as with blisters. Particularly noticeable from friction of food when eating.
12.30.4.18:00
My tongue feels raw and sore.
5.200.11
Small, painful lesions in my mouth, lower right side.
7.30.15
Blisters in my mouth are getting worse. Irritation of the whole area, < after eating a tangerine.
10.30.1.6:40
Very dry mouth on waking, not improved after brushing teeth.

White - Coated
2.200.0.16:00
My tongue is thin and has a white coating at the base, and the side, at the front.

Burning - Numb
1.30.0.7:35
A burning sensation starting under the right half of the tongue, only the area at the front initially.
1.30.0.9:45

Distension of the whole side and underneath part of the right side of the tongue, with no visible change.

By midday the burning sensation had changed to numbness, then during the course of the day this moves to the area underneath the back of the tongue (right).

1.30.1

A small numb area at the side of the tongue, underneath on the right, which lasts until the end of the day.

<u>Salivation</u>

2.200.4.15:00

Extreme salivation following afternoon nap (large wet patch), and I feel frozen and am sneezing.

6.30.27

The dry mouth has gone, instead of that I constantly feel that saliva is dribbling from the corner of my mouth (which is not the case). This sensation lasted for a week altogether.

10.30.0.10:40

Increased salivation and dribbling when I lie on my side.

<u>Biting</u>

10.30.10.9.00

I have noticed that my fingertips are dry. Tiny bits of skin are peeling away at the tip of the index finger.

I catch myself biting them off.

<u>Pressure</u>

2.200.0.16:00

Pressure pain parotid gland right and somewhat in left.

<u>Tingling</u>

2.200.0.21:00

Mild tingling in gums.

Teeth

<u>Sensitive to heat</u>

10.30.22.17:00

All my teeth are sensitive to heat.

<u>Pulling sensation - As if inflamed</u>

11.30.11.13:00

Ground to a halt by midday and need to have a lie-down. Feels like the flu, with some pressure in my left ear.
Also pressure in my head (forehead and skull) and eyes, with drawing sensation in the upper left molars.
11.30.13
Blocked nose with no discharge. Left nostril feels very dry. Left upper molars are very painful, as with maxillary sinusitis. Feel like I've got flu, but no fever.

Throat

Burning - Stabbing - Numb
2.200.0.16:00
Stabbing pain in my heart.
Warm hands and face.
Sore throat, mild burning.
2.200.0.16:30
Stabbing pains in left tonsil, only on the left side.
2.200.0.21:00
Pharynx red, mild burning.
Burning and numbness in pharynx, as if slightly anaesthetised.
2.200.10.4.00
Mild burning in throat.
2.200.21
Mild angina in the morning, right side, pricking?? sensation. 38.0 fever, perspiration at night, all symptoms has disappeared by midday.
3.30.3
Mild stabbing in throat, particularly right side.
3.30.4
Stabbing in throat sometimes distinct, sometimes absent.

Congested with phlegm
11.30.19
Nose and pharynx severely congested with phlegm overnight, and I had to blow out and cough up large amounts of yellow to clear phlegm.

Full of cold air
12.30.4.18:00
Urge to cough with sensation as if my throat was full of cold air.

Stomach

Nausea - Queasy - Vomiting - Urge to vomit - Pressure
1.30.2
Slight problems with circulation in the morning felt as mild nausea, particularly when travelling on public transport.
1.30.19.17:00
Poor circulation: debility, shaky legs, mild nausea, blurred vision, < sitting.
3.30.19
Queasy feeling in my stomach on getting up, eased by fennel tea and grated apple.
3.30.19
Depressed, Queasy feeling, > after walking in the fresh air.
5.200.4
Mild nausea, self doubt and feel tired and worn out. Am very absent-minded.
8.Plac.0.17:00
Mild pressure in my head behind my forehead and eyes, comes and goes.
Also mild nausea. Feels like the nausea is connected to the metallic taste I am experiencing.
8.Plac.4.19:00
Nausea again and an unpleasant taste in my mouth. And I can't stand any external pressure on my stomach.
11.30.11
Nausea building up after breakfast, triggered by black tea.
Feel somewhat light-headed generally.
3.30.18
Vomiting, the vomit gets into the paranasal sinuses, and from there tingling and stabbing pains which extend to the head, especially the vertex.
The nausea comes on in sudden fits (vomited 4 times), I can't even keep water down.
2.200.0.17:15
Pressure pain in abdomen, initially for a very short time on the right, then only on the left for a short time.
Queasy feeling in the stomach area, passing copious amounts of wind.
12.30.3.8:00
Nausea while brushing teeth, which I had only ever experienced before during pregnancy.
Ravenous hunger.
10.30.14.13:00
I feel ravenous again.
Thirst for water
1.30.2.12:00
Intense thirst, sudden onset. I had to drink cold water immediately, a lot of it and quickly.

Abdomen

Hollow and empty
10.30.1.6:40
Mild vertigo and empty sensation in my abdomen when standing in front of the wash-basin.
10.30.13
A hollow sensation in the whole of the large intestine area, particularly on the right side in the ascending colon (lasts about 2 hours).
10.30.14.10:00
Empty sensation in abdomen. I absolutely have to eat a second breakfast.

Tension and pressure - electric shock
11.30.6
I bought a packet of mixed Haribo (fruit flavoured sweets with liquorice) and make my way to the motorway. The sweets don't taste right and give me a distended abdomen.
11.30.13.18:00
Pressure pain in the left hip-bone.
12.30.0.
Flatulence developing during the morning.
12.30.0.8:00
Sensation like electric shocks in right ear after the first dose of the remedy, a couple of times in a row.
One minute later I notice the same sensation in the upper abdomen, but somewhat weaker.

Itching, making we want to scratch
10.30.7
Itch, making me want to scratch my abdomen. Pale pink discolouration, an area the size of a 5 Mark piece, just above the pubic hair and it itches like a mosquito bite (but how could that happen in November?).

Rectum

Passing copious amounts of wind
2.200.0.17:15
Pressure pain in abdomen, initially for a very short time on the right, then only on the left for a short time.
Queasy feeling in the stomach area, passing copious amounts of wind.
2.200.1.14:00

84

Short and intense passing of wind following lunch (I never have this after eating green beans usually).

Haemorrhoids - Bleeding - Wind
6.30.3
Woke in the night with strong haemorrhoid pain, pressing from inside out. Lying on my abdomen > the pain.
6.30.50
My haemorrhoid complaint has disappeared. I last experienced this 12 years ago!!
10.30.3.23:00
First dragging in the bowels here and there, then diarrhoea, mixture of runny and firm. Followed by bleeding haemorrhoids and a sore feeling in the rectum.

Stool

Light brown - mixture of firm and runny
6.30.1.14:30
Light brown diarrhoea an hour after lunch, runny.
10.30.3.23:00
First dragging in the bowels back and forth, then diarrhoea, mixture of runny and firm. Followed by bleeding haemorrhoids and a sore feeling in the rectum.

Light brown
6.30.1.14:30
Light brown diarrhoea an hour after lunch, runny.

Bladder

Pressure and full feeling - Cramp and retention
1.30.8.
Permanent pressure on the bladder, but not causing frequent urination (lasting until I fell asleep).
1.30.9
The abdominal twinges and the pressure on the bladder from the day before remain unchanged and last until the evening again.
1.30.10
The abdominal twinges and the pressure on the bladder remain unchanged until the late afternoon when they disappear with the onset of menses.
10.30.22.5:30

I wake and need to urinate. It is difficult for me to let go even though my bladder is very full. It seems to me that the involuntary muscles block one another. It takes a while before I am able to urinate. Then there is pain in the sphincter muscle, like cramp.

11.30.12

It's still dark when I wake up. My bladder is full and my penis erect, which prevents me from falling asleep again. I have to empty my bladder so that I can fall asleep again. The same thing happened to me the last 2 nights.

11.30.12

Sleep until 4.00 am and wake again with a full bladder and erect penis.
Have to go to the toilet again to empty my bladder.

Urge in the night - Empty feeling

10.30.8

I have noticed that I have had to get up almost every night to urinate (very unusual). After urinating I have a totally empty feeling in my abdomen.

Kidney

Pressure - Stabbing

2.200.1.7:30

Brief sensation of pressure in my left kidney.

2.200.1.10:00

Stabbing in left kidney, stabbing in back, right kidney.

2.200.2.10:45

Severe pressure in left kidney, initially with mild stabbing.

2.200.3.15:00

Pressure pain in left kidney.

2.200.7.16:00

Pressure pain in left kidney.

Urethra

Pressure - Letting go - Cramped

10.30.22.5:30

I wake and need to urinate. It is difficult for me to let go even though my bladder is very full. It seems to me that the involuntary muscles block one another. It takes a while before I am able to urinate. Then there is pain in the sphincter muscle, like cramp.

86

Female Genitalia

Stabbing - Stitching - sometimes right, sometimes left - like a band
1.30.8.
Abdominal pain since waking, stitching, short duration, one after the other, sometimes in the right ovary, sometimes the left (lasting until I fell asleep).
1.30.9
The abdominal stitches and the pressure on the bladder from the day before remain unchanged and last until the evening again.
1.30.10
The abdominal stitches and the pressure on the bladder remain unchanged until the late afternoon when they disappear with the onset of menses.
2.200.1.9:30
Mild stitches in my lower abdomen (ovaries?), starting off mild, right sided, then very noticeable on the left side, with stabbing pain in my right temple simultaneously, then wandering, stabbing pain in my forehead.
2.200.1.14:00
Intermittent stitches in right ovary for the last 3 days.
6.30.4.11:30
Mild dragging pain in both ovaries, < right side, gone after 15 minutes. The pain dragged like a band from one side to the other.

Pressure from inside outwards - Congestion -
No flow during the night - Profuse flow during the night
1.30.12.8:00
Woken as a result of menstrual symptoms; dragging pain in abdomen from inside outwards, with nausea making me feel I'd have to vomit. I had the feeling that the menstrual blood had clogged up inside me and wasn't going to flow freely, and I actually didn't lose any blood that night. Restlessness, moving around here and there in the flat, trying to find a position in which I could tolerate this incredible pain.
1.30.12.9:00
The abdominal dragging pain has subsided somewhat, still coming on throughout the day, sometimes stronger, sometimes less, as also the weariness and tiredness.
6.30.12
Menses flowing only during the daytime.
6.30.50
Menses 10 days late. Once again only flowing during the day, ceasing during the night.
9.Plac.14
Unusually profuse menstrual bleeding, to the extent that blood seeped through to my knickers and pyjamas.

Wave-like - Increasing - Decreasing
1.30.13
still getting the abdominal pains from the previous day, increasing and decreasing in waves, until late afternoon when they cease of their own accord, for no apparent reason.

Itching - Dry - Open - Aversion
2.200.2.22:00
Mild itching in the vagina again in the evening. As a result of this a very pleasant feeling during sex, linked with a lot of affection, talking and openness.
12.30.7.
Absolutely no desire for sex at present, especially due to painful vaginal dryness.

Late
12.30.18
Menses a week late, usually exactly four week intervals.

Brown thread - String
3.30.3
Very little menstrual blood, dark brown threads.
Then increase in whitish-brown discharge.
3.30.6
I notice a dried thread of blood, like string, in my knickers and a bit of a brown discharge.
6.30.13
Menses: Bright red blood, contains a lot of dark bits of mucous membrane.

Bleeding after having a bath
3.30.25
Menses really kicks in after having a bath.

Male genitalia

Erections during the night
11.30.12
It's still dark when I wake up. My bladder is full and my penis erect, which prevents me from falling asleep again. I have to empty my bladder so that I can fall asleep again. The same thing happened to me the last 2 nights.

88

11.30.12
Sleep until 4.00 am and wake again with a full bladder and erect penis.
Have to go to the toilet again to empty my bladder.

<u>Pressure in the prostate during the night</u>
11.30.28
Wake with intense pain (pressing, stabbing) in my prostate, just above the pubic bone (after coition). The pain is very unpleasant and lasts the whole day.

Cough

<u>Dry - Barking</u>
2.200.2.7:00
The dry cough continues to loosen up.
2.200.7.7:00
The dry cough has been about 80% better for a few days.
11.30.19.16:00
My cough is getting worse. It is a terrible barking cough, and comes on very suddenly. The urge to cough comes on in isolated bouts, abruptly, no matter what I am doing at the time.
The cough is < when lying down, lying one my back, and doing anything physical.

<u>Cough (urge to) - Pepper - Chilli - Water</u>
11.30.21
Relentless cough after eating a Turkish dish containing chilli. Not eased by drinking water.
11.30.27
Strong urge to cough after eating freshly ground pepper.
12.30.4.18:00
Urge to cough with sensation as if my throat was full of cold air.

Expectoration

<u>Yellow expectoration</u>
11.30.19
Nose and pharynx severely congested with phlegm overnight, and I had to blow out and cough up large amounts of yellow to clear phlegm.

Chest

Stabbing - Trapped - Pressure
1.30.7
A stabbing pain in right side of chest as if a nerve was trapped. It came on after waking, lasting until I went to sleep. The pain is centred around the front and extends through the chest backwards, > inhaling.
2.200.0.16:00
Stabbing pain in my heart.
Warm hands and face.
Sore throat, mild burning.
2.200.1.7:30
Mild palpitation, stabbing in the heart (for about 10 minutes)
11.30.7.10:00
Vertigo from my ears upwards (not in the whole of my head) after getting up from the chair.
Pressure in my left breast lasting approximately 10 seconds, it comes and goes. I am somewhat concerned. Nothing has an effect on it.
11.30.13.18:00
I am conscious of my eyes, they feel hot, but I don't have any fever. Feeling of tension in the bronchial tubes and lungs.

Chilliness
10.30.0.11:10
Sudden chilliness in left breast (disappears just as quick).
Cold ears (noticed it suddenly).

Palpitation
2.200.0.13:00
Palpitation for about 20 minutes.
2.200.3.7:00
Violent palpitation on waking.

Itching - Chapped - Sore
1.30.2.21:00
Sudden, intense itching on sternum, > scratching intensely for a long time.
1.30.3.10:00
This is the third time I've had the urge to scratch my breastbone.
2.200.1.14:00
Moist right nipple, sensitive when bathing.
2.200.2.7:00

90

Very sensitive right nipple, itching.
2.200.3.8:00
Intense itching under the left axilla (inner side, towards the breast), red after scratching. A small patch, dark red, like eczema.
6.30.39
Skin under my breast has been really dry and flaky for 4 days (like bran flakes), no pain or itching.
12.30.5.9:00
While I was showering I noticed a brown mark, the size of my thumb, near my axilla, looks like a café-au-lait mark, not painful.
12.30.12
I noticed some pimples on my left breast in the evening. They are red and itch a lot when touched. The glands around the areola have increased in size and protrude like small nodules.

Back

<u>Sore muscles</u>
1.30.3
The whole of my back has felt like I pulled a muscle for the whole of the day, from my neck, including the area at the back of my shoulder to the lumbar area, > keeping still.

<u>Compressed together - Pressure</u>
1.30.15
Sudden, severe pain in the lumbar area when lifting a heavy box with books in. It feels as if my spine has been compressed together and the individual vertebrae are out of alignment. I experience tremendous pain and stiffness when I move.
10.30.23.8:00
Slipped on steps and banged my left buttock. Feeling of compression in my back.
1.30.16.11:00
After sitting a while (45 minute train journey) the pain has suddenly disappeared with just mild lumbar pressure remaining.
10.30.5.8:00
The pain in the sacral area has returned, better for pressure (fist or flat hand), also > from lying on the painful part (lying flat on the back).

<u>Motion - Rest - Bending</u>
1.30.13
Mild lumbar pain lasting throughout the whole day, > from resting.
10.30.0.9:55

My back is so incredibly painful, not improved by motion (as is usually the case).
10.30.5.8:30
The sacral pain is < bending forward, also < putting on trousers.
11.30.11
Lumbar pain (L3-L4). Lancinating and < bending forward.
Really exhausted around 9.00 pm and have to go to bed. I make sure I don't lie on my back as this aggravates the pain in my back.
11.30.13.
Feel full of cold and ill.
Lumbar pains are very intense after getting up. They are < bending down and after getting up from a chair. When I bend forward I get the lancinating pain again, with the feeling that I'm going to snap in two .
10.30.2.14:30
Remittent back pain, especially when I have been crouching in one position for a while on the floor with the children
Carrying
11.30.13.14:00
Lumbar pain extending to both hips when carrying a tray.

Light - Wine
10.30.4.20.15
Back pain has disappeared after 3 glasses of wine (I had pain in the sacral area all day).
10.30.6.8:00
This is the first morning that I have woken with no back pain. Everything is getting easier.

Weak - Paralysis
10.30.3.11:30
Weakness in the lumbar region, extending to sacrum, after housework.
10.30.10.9:00
The back pain is in the background all the time, but doesn't bother me as much, it is more like a paralysis.

Stabbing
2.200.1.10:00
Stabbing in left kidney, stabbing pain in the back, right kidney.

Itching
10.30.21.21:00
Intense itching on my back from 9.00 pm.

Extremities

Pumped up - Don't belong to me - Twisted - Pulled

1.30.1
My knees feel like they don't belong to my body, a little like they had been pumped up, not painful.
6.30.0.13:30
Left knee feels like it's been twisted, < walking, < bending (when driving).
7.30.3.8:00
Dragging in my right shoulder and sensation as if I'd pulled a muscle since waking up; < lifting up my arm when moving backwards. Feel as if I have to make a counter movement to ease the pain, but it doesn't help.

Weak - Heavy - Shaky - Dropping things
1.30.19.17:00
Poor circulation: debility, shaky legs, mild nausea, blurred vision, < sitting.
10.30.0.10:40
Dropped the post
10.30.1.6:40
I still have really heavy limbs at breakfast time.

Battered - Bruised
12.30.10
During the night shift I constantly had the feeling that the muscles that are normally compressed when sitting, had gone to sleep (especially the thigh). My muscles feel bruised generally.

Dry - Cracked - Itchy - Small blisters - Peeling - Leprosy
1.30.15.20:00
Sudden appearance of redness and dry skin on the middle and front finger joints on both hands at around 10.00 pm. Outbreaks in various places on my skin within an hour and there are small lesions that burn.
1.30. 16
Finger joints continue to be red, dry and cracked.
3.30.3
Itching on the inside of the elbow in the evening.
3.30.4
Right elbow itching from time to time, better after a good scratch
3.30.4
Elbow is itching in the same place again in the evening, scratching doesn't help much.

3.30.7
Increased itching in the elbow, cold water >, having a good scratch >.
3.30.10
Feet itching incredibly after dinner, when warming up (had felt frozen the whole of the day until then).
6.30.2.
Itching and suppuration of small blisters filled with water between 3rd and 4th toe on right foot, painful after scratching, having a shower >.
9.Plac.21
I have developed a wart on my right foot, under the left toe.
10.30.10.9.00
I have noticed that my fingertips are dry. Tiny bits of skin are peeling away at the tip of the index finger.
I catch myself biting them off.
10.30.14.20:00
The skin on my fingertips is pealing again.
11.30.0.7:30
Large blisters, itchy and filled with water on left index finger on the inside (I am not at all happy about this because I don't want to have a skin complaint!)
11.30.0.21:00
I can feel a water-filled blister (index finger). I don't pay any more attention to it. Only hope I won't catch leprosy.

Cramp
12.30.8
Cramps in right thigh when lying on my left side and vice versa on the left side when lying on my right.

Warm - Cold
2.200.0.8:00
Warm hands
2.200.0.10:00
Warm hands and tired eyes.
2.200.0.16:00
Stabbing pain in my heart.
Warm hands and face.
Sore throat, mild burning.
2.200.0.19:00
Hands are very warm.
Warm face.

2.200.1.14:00
Warm hands and face.
2.200.2.16:00
Generally warmer than usual, most noticeable on hands and face.

2.200.10.18:00
Felt frozen until 5.00 pm. Now I am lovely and warm, especially my hands and face.
10.30.14.20:00
Feet very hot in the evening. Felt very warm the whole of the day, even though everyone else thinks it's very cold today.
10.30.16.12:00
Hot flushes on the upper part of my body, and my right foot feels cold.
12.30.0.20:00
Hands and feet have been cold all the time.

Swollen - Stiff - Blue
10.30.25
Wake in the night with stiffness in my hands, which disappears quickly after movement. The stiffness continues to be present every time I wake up
12.30.1.
My hands are swollen and stiff.
12.30.2
My hands are swollen and stiff again today.
10.30.16.12:00
Feels like there's a bruise on my shin (but nothing's visible), painful to touch.

Pains in the limbs

Stabbing - Sharp knife
3.30.13
Stabbing pain, where the skin is open, under the right middle toe. The stabbing pain comes on from movement and touch, sharp like a knife.

Pressing
1.30.0.14:45
Pain in both knees just above the patella, stronger on the left than the right. Sensation: just a light pressing pain and only when bending the lower leg 90°. The areas are sensitive to pressure, < from warmth.
6.30.0.14:30

Pressure pain left hip on the outer side.

Dull - Open Window - Shoulder - Driving a car
3.30.5
Dull pain in right shoulder joint when lying on it. I slept under an open window last night, which could have been the trigger.
The pain disappeared once I was up.
9.Plac.0.10.05
Pain in left shoulder joint, extending to my upper arm (when driving) and gone after the drive.

Thumbs - Writing
9.Plac.19
Pain in my thumb knuckle while writing.

Sleep

Unrefreshing - Bad - Deep
1.30.1
Unrefreshing sleep, waking frequently in the night, no dreams.
10.30.8
Incredibly tired in the morning, despite a long, undisturbed sleep.
11.30.20
Poor sleep in the last couple of nights is taking it out on me somewhat. I am not as energetic and have to have a rest more often.
1.30.13
Deep and sound sleep, but not so refreshing.
1.30.3
Deep, sound sleep, with no dreams, interrupted once by the recurring itch on the sternum, which woke me.

Tossing and turning - Restless
1.30.3
Difficulty falling asleep, tossing and turning. Unwelcomed, worrying thoughts about present circumstances come into my mind. After about an hour I have a compulsive need to open the window wide open, feel I need to breathe in fresh air, which makes me feel better and I can then fall asleep.
1.30.4
Restless sleep with several interruptions.
Towards morning a dream definitely touching on one of the themes in my life at present regarding

96

conflict
Feeling in the dream: Panic, desperation, helplessness.
5.200.1
Woke up several times in the night.

<u>Wide awake - Awake</u>
6.30.1.6:00
Hear my husband's alarm (usually never or seldom), am wide awake, but fall back asleep again easily.
6.30.1.7:00
Woken by my daughter, am awake straight away, can get up easily.

<u>Four o'clock - One and two o'clock</u>
11.30.14
Woke at 4 am again. Difficult to get back to sleep again this time. On top of this my nose was completely blocked.
5.200.11
I have been waking between 1.30 and 2.30 am on a regular basis with problems in my head to do with circulation, which frighten me. I get out of bed, feel like I've drunk a lot of alcohol. Feel dizzy, then I get back to bed again, calm myself down and am able to fall asleep again.

Chill

2.200.3.17:00
Very cold, nervous.
2.200.4.15:00
Extreme salivation following afternoon nap (large wet patch), and I feel frozen and am sneezing.
10.30.23.17:00
Heat in my head, yet feeling cold in my body, feel slightly chilly.
11.30.13
Feel freezing cold and dress up warm in the flat.

Perspiration

<u>Night sweats</u>
2.200.2.7:00
Woke drenched in sweat, my whole body is clammy.
2.200.8.9:00

Strong night sweat on whole body.
2.200.21
Mild angina in the morning, right side, possibly a pricking sensation. Rectal temperature 38.0°, perspiration at night, all symptoms have disappeared by midday.

Skin

Itching - Scratching - Dry
1.30.2.21:00
Sudden, intense itching on sternum, > scratching intensely for a long time.
3.30.4
Elbow is itching in the same place again in the evening, scratching doesn't help much.
6.30.0.21:00
Itching of an old scar (gall bladder operation).
12.30.8
Extremely dry skin generally.

Cold water
3.30.7
Increased itching in the elbow, cold water >, having a good scratch >.

Leprosy - Small blisters
11.30.0.7:30
Large blisters, itchy and filled with water on left index finger on the inside (I am not at all happy about this because I don't want to have a skin condition!)
11.30.0.21:00
I can feel a water-filled blister (index finger). I don't pay any more attention to it. Only hope I won't catch leprosy.

Café-au-lait
12.30.5.9:00
While I was showering I noticed a brown mark, the size of my thumb, near my axilla, looks like a café-au-lait mark, not painful.

98

Generalities

Tired - Weak - Slow - Heavy

1.30.2

Slight problems with circulation in the morning felt as mild nausea, particularly when travelling on public transport.

1.30.2.12:00

Considerable tiredness throughout the whole day, weary down to the bones, physically as well as psychologically.

1.30.2.21:30

Had to go to bed straight away and fell asleep instantly.

1.30.4.17:00

Intense tiredness and weariness which came on suddenly.

1.30.5

Sudden onset of tiredness.

1.30.8.17:00

Considerable tiredness, came on suddenly.

1.30.12.9:00

Fell asleep again and didn't wake until 2.00 pm. Feel weary, drained with a similar feeling to when you wake up in the morning with a fever.

The abdominal dragging pain has subsided somewhat, still coming on throughout the day, sometimes stronger, sometimes less, as also the weariness and tiredness.

1.30.18

Feel very tired as if I haven't had enough sleep.

1.30.19

Very tired and heavy.

1.30.19.17:00

Poor circulation: debility, shaky legs, mild nausea, blurred vision, < sitting.

1.30.20

Very tired, heavy.

1.30.21

Very tired, heavy.

1.30.22

Very tired and heavy.

2.200.1.7:30

Feel very tired, would prefer not to have to go to work.

2.200.8.13:00

Not able to concentrate at work and exhausted.

I feel very tired at midday, also still exhausted after an afternoon nap.

2.200.9.10:00

I slept for a long time, but feel very exhausted, not capable of concentrating on my work. I would prefer not to have to do anything at all and flap (like a chicken) between the kitchen and the office without accomplishing much.

Strong feelings of grief again, the first time since taking the remedy, feels more like a paralysis of energy.

2.200.9.17:00

Feeling exhausted before and after midday nap. I am shocked that the day is almost over.

8.Plac.0.9:00

I feel very tired and weary, no energy. I could fall asleep while sitting even though I went to bed early yesterday.

10.30.0.10:40

Slept well for half an hour, I'm absolutely shattered.

10.30.0.10:40

Tiredness has become even worse after sleeping.

10.30.1.6:40

It takes me a while to get going.

10.30.2.18.00

The light feeling is dwindling.

10.30.3.6:40

It's taking me a long time to wake up today.

I've got the impression it's taking me a long time getting things done this morning.

10.30.17.10:45

Tiredness (like lead) at the desk at work. I even fell asleep bent forward.

10.30.23.18:30

Feel old and stiff.

11.30.12

I feel ill and yet not ill. It's very strange. In spite of everything I can do almost everything, but just slower.

11.30.20

The poor sleep in the last couple of nights is taking it out on me somewhat. I am not as energetic and have to have a rest more often.

12.30.0.10:00

Try to read a book. But I keep falling asleep all the time. On one occasion I wake up with such a terrible shock, that a violent jerk goes right through me.

Battered - Bruised

12.30.10

During the night shift I constantly had the feeling that the muscles that are normally compressed when sitting had gone to asleep (especially the thigh). My muscles feel bruised generally.

12.30.12

100

When falling asleep on my side (my favourite position) as soon as the muscles are compressed from lying on them they go to sleep. And with this the beaten and crushed feeling again.

Full of energy - Young - Beautiful
2.200.8.13:00
Full of energy again at the dance course and am enjoying learning.
2.200.10.9.00
A lot of energy and in the mood for work despite feeling like I've got a cold.
2.200.10.18:00
I'm astonished that I feel full of energy, despite feeling like I've got a cold. Can work and am very focused.
5.200.5
A lot of people have said that I look different (look younger).
5.200.17
A lot of people have said I look younger. Things are not affecting me as much at the moment, more able to distance myself from things.
9.Plac.0.13:05
Am not tired at all, in high spirits, usually I am always tired after work. I'm very surprised about this.
11.30.5
I am sitting in a seminar and thinking about how much homeopathy changes people. It makes them beautiful - in a unique way - and young.

Accidents
2.200.10.10.00
Cut my left index finger badly with the bread knife.
2.200.27
My daughter's birthday. Another accident: I actually feel that I don't have any more proving symptoms. But because it possibly fits in with the concept to do with the bread knife and the dream about a knife I have written it down.
I was cooking 2 chickens in a large pressure cooker that I don't normally use. I also have a smaller, one which needs to be opened in a different way to release the steam.
My mother had put the lid on, the pressure is at it's highest when I open it, using force, thinking that the lid has jammed (as is frequently the case with the smaller pressure cooker). Then the chickens shoot out up to the ceiling and I scald my back and hairline badly with the hot steam and stock.
I don't normally have accidents of this kind, and generally tend to be more on the cautious side.
5.200.65
After dreaming that my tom-cat had a fall (belly flop) I fall when coming out of a friend's front door. I've grazed and bruised myself and I'm in a lot of pain. My purse has fallen under a car. I

pick up all my things and spend the whole evening lying on the sofa with my cat. My thoughts about this: I am getting old. I was talking about the Fountain of Youth and themes to do with addiction today. I will have to keep moving, otherwise I will cease up.

9.Plac.3.7:20

I rub my eye in such an awkward fashion that I poke my eyeball, which has caused some irritation to the eye.

9.Plac.18.8:15

Bang myself on the cupboard and bruise my right upper arm.
Shortly after, I burn my right index finger with hot oil.

9.Plac.23

Give myself a paper cut on the left thumb.

9.Plac.30

Cut myself on the right index finger.

10.30.18.17:45

Almost caused an accident on the way home after going to the farmer's. It was dark and I didn't see a delivery van coming from the left side. Only just missed it by the skin of my teeth. Where did it come from?

10.30.23.8:00

Slipped on steps and banged my left buttock. Feeling of compression in my back.

Desire - Aversion

1.30.2.12:00

Intense thirst, sudden onset. I had to drink cold water immediately, a lot of it and quickly.

5.200.66

I keep wanting to take the remedy.

6.30.6.15:00

Extremely strong craving for coffee.
I went to see '7 Years in Tibet' at the cinema in the evening. I am deeply impressed with how Peter Harrer sheds his tough exterior.

10.30.3.13:00

Suddenly had a craving for cold milk while cooking. Then had 3 large glasses of milk before lunch.

10.30.4.20.15

Back pain has disappeared after 3 glasses of wine (I had pain in the sacral area all day).

11.30.6

What has been striking in the last two days is a strong thirst for tea, which I have given into with relish.

11.30.6

I bought a packet of mixed Haribo (fruit flavoured sweets with liquorice) and make my way to the motorway. The sweets don't taste right and give me a distended abdomen.

11.30.8

102

I continue to notice my extreme thirst for black tea.

11.30.13

Aversion to cigarette smoke. I am frequently overcome with a peculiar feeling of abhorrence, yet I experience pity when I see others smoking. It is really evident to me how addiction eats away at people. Probably a more intense feeling because I was once into asceticism.

11.30.13

Sensation of heat internally, particularly in the mouth and pharynx, urethra, stomach and eyes, with a desire for cold water.

But I only drink a little as my body often feels frozen and would prefer not to have to go out before or after 11.00 am to 4.00 pm.

6.30.25

I can't be bothered writing more of the same stuff down. I'm going to have another coffee!!!!

Calm - Warm
2.200.4.7:00

Feel warm, very calm.

2.200.6

Feel calmer again and warm.

Fresh air
1.30.3

Difficulty falling asleep, tossing and turning. Unwelcomed, worrying thoughts about present circumstances come into my mind. After about an hour I have a compulsive need to open the window wide open, feel I need to breathe in fresh air, which makes me feel better and I can then fall asleep.

Alternating between dreams and physical symptoms
10.30.13

It feels like the dreams are alternating with the physical symptoms. There are few physical symptoms on days following copious dreams and vice versa there are many symptoms following nights in which there has been little dream recall.

As if symptoms
1.30.1

My knees feel like they don't belong to my body, a little like they had been pumped up, not painful.

5.200.37

I am becoming more decisive, I re-experience emotional connections from the past with great clarity, as if a curtain had been pulled aside.

9.Plac.0.9:55

Feeling as if someone else was fastening my shoelaces.

10.30.8.9:30

Throughout the day I keep getting the feeling that I hadn't washed my face today.
6.30.27

The dry mouth has gone, instead of that I constantly feel that saliva is dribbling from the corner of my mouth (but which is not the case). This sensation lasted for a week altogether.
12.30.4.18:00

Urge to cough with sensation as if my throat was full of cold air.
10.30.14.

Dream

I am at university. We are sitting in class being taught, I think it's maths. All of a sudden I have to cough. I want to get a lozenge out of my bag. My bag is a complete mess, lots of pens and sweets, and everything falls out of my bag, which disrupts the class quite a bit. There's a splashing sound coming from the benches behind me as if someone is having a pee.

Repertory Additions *[P.K. & J.W.]*

W Weißwein   **R Rotwein**   **N** (new symptom in repertory!)   **C** (clinical)

MIND; ACTIVITY (SI-8) (159) **W** **R**

MIND; AILMENTS from; anger, vexation; suppressed, from (K2, SI-15, G2) (23)
W

MIND; ANGER, irascibility; tendency (K2, SI-26, G1) (308) **W**

MIND; ANGER, irascibility; tendency; sudden (SI-37) (11) **W**

MIND; COMMUNICATIVE, expansive (SI-144) (10) **R**

MIND; CONFUSION of mind (K13, SI-160, G11) (395) **R**

MIND; CONFUSION of mind; concentrate the mind, on attempting to (K14, SI-167, G12) (14) **R**

MIND; DELUSIONS, imaginations; body, body parts; knees pumped up (1) **R** **N**

MIND; DELUSIONS, imaginations; walls; moving towards her (1) **W** **N**

MIND; DREAMS; accidents, of (K1235, SIII-241, G1020) (43) **W** **R**

MIND; DREAMS; animals, of (K1236, SIII-247, G1020) (120) **W** **R**

MIND; DREAMS; animals, of; badger (1) **W** **N**

MIND; DREAMS; animals, of; biting him (K1236, SIII-255, G1020) (15) **W**

MIND; DREAMS; animals, of; horses (K1240, SIII-311, G1024) (30) **R**

MIND; DREAMS; confused (K1237, SIII-268, G1021) (131) **W**

MIND; DREAMS; cutting; knife, being cut with a (K1237, SIII-272,G1021) (5) **R**

MIND; DREAMS; family, own (SIII-298) (5) **W** **R**

MIND; DREAMS; feasting (K1239, SIII-299, G1023) (11) **W**

MIND; DREAMS; hurried (K1241, SIII-313, G1024) (7) **W**

MIND; DREAMS; journey (K1241, SIII-316, G1024) (60) **R**

MIND; DREAMS; mutilation (K1242, SIII-326, G1025) (11) **R**

MIND; DREAMS; pursued, of being (K1242, SIII-337, G1025) (27) **W**

MIND; DREAMS; relatives (SIII-340) (3) **W**

MIND; DREAMS; restless (SIII-342) (54) **W**

MIND; DREAMS; riding (SIII-343) (7) **R**

MIND; IRRITABILITY (K57, SI-653, G46) (493) **W**

MIND; MISTAKES, makes; time, in (K66, SI-177, SI-749, G53) (43) **R**

MIND; RESPONSIBILITY; strong (17) **C**

MIND; SLOWNESS (K81, SI-930, G65) (91) **W** **R**

MIND; STUPEFACTION, as if intoxicated (K84, SI-966, G67) (272) **W** **R**

MIND; STUPEFACTION, as if intoxicated; cotton, as if in (1) **W** **R** **N**

MIND; TRANQUILLITY, serenity, calmness (K89, SI-1029, G71) (110) **W**

MIND; WEEPING, tearful mood; tendency (K92, SI-1066, G74) (357) **W**
MIND; WEEPING, tearful mood; tendency; trifles, at (K94, SI-1089, G76) (40) **W**

VERTIGO; VERTIGO (K96, G79) (365) **W** **R**
VERTIGO; GROUND gives way, as if (11) **W** **R**
VERTIGO; OBJECTS seem; move, to; fixed, when (1) **W** **N**

HEAD PAIN; FOREIGN BODY, as if (K186, G154) (6) **W**
HEAD PAIN; PRESSING (K188, G157) (385) **W** **R**

EYE; PAIN; foreign body, as from (K256, G215) (119) **R**
VISION; FOGGY (K279, G235) (188) **R**

EAR; ITCHING in (K291, G245) (183) **R**
EAR; PAIN; electric, like electric sparks (1) **W** **R** **N**

FACE; CRACKS; corners of mouth (K357, G301) (49) **R**
FACE; DRYNESS; lips (K364, G307) (177) **R**
FACE; ERUPTIONS; herpes; lips (K369, G310) (69) **R**
FACE; HEAT; cheeks (G319) (21) **R**
FACE; PAIN; burnt, as if (8) **W**

MOUTH; DISCOLORATION; redness; gums; margins bright red
    (K400,G339)(5) **W**
MOUTH; DRYNESS (K403, G341) (337) **W**
MOUTH; DRYNESS; thirst, with (K403, G342) (69) **W**
MOUTH; ERUPTIONS; vesicles (K429, G364) (131) **W**
MOUTH; ERUPTIONS; vesicles; sore, smarting (K429, G364) (5) **W**
MOUTH; INFLAMMATION; sore spots (1) **W** **R** **N**
MOUTH; PAIN; burning, raw, smarting; numbness, with (1) **R** **N**
MOUTH; PAIN; sore (K413, G350) (222) **W** **R**
MOUTH; SALIVATION; running out of mouth (1) **R** **N**

TEETH; CONSCIOUSNESS of teeth (1) **W** **N**
TEETH, LOOSENESS of; sensation; biting teeth together; amel. (1) **W** **N**
TEETH; PAIN; General; biting teeth together; amel. (K435, G371) (25) **W**

THROAT; DRYNESS (K450, G383) (293) **W**
THROAT; DRYNESS; thirst; with (8) **W**
THROAT; PAIN; burning; numbness, with (1) **R** **N**

STOMACH; NAUSEA; morning (K505, G430) (148) **R**
STOMACH; RETCHING, gagging; brushing teeth (2) **R**
STOMACH; UNEASINESS (K531, G447) (76) **R**

ABDOMEN; DISTENSION; constipation, during (K545, G464) (16) **W**
ABDOMEN; DISTENSION; sweets, after (1) **R N**
ABDOMEN; KNOTTED sensation (14) **W**

RECTUM; FLATUS (K617, G527) (273) **W**
RECTUM; FLATUS; loud (K618, G528) (42) **W**
RECTUM; FLATUS; offensive (K618, G528) (148) **W**
RECTUM; HEMORRHOIDS (K619, G530) (258) **R**
RECTUM; PAIN; pressing, pressure; hemorrhoids, with (5) **R**

BLADDER; FULLNESS, sensation of; erections, with (1) **R N**
BLADDER; PAIN; pressing, pressure in; menses, before (1) **R N**
BLADDER; URGING to urinate, morbid desire; night (K652, G558) (120) **R**

URETHRA; TENESMUS; urination. after (1) **R N**

MALE; ERECTIONS, troublesome; waking him (3) **R**

FEMALE; DRYNESS; Vagina (K717, G612) (30) **R**
FEMALE; ITCHING; Vagina (K720, G614) (71) **R**
FEMALE; MENSES; General; daytime only (K724, SIII-520, G617) (16) **R**
FEMALE; MENSES; late, too (K727, SIII-547, G619) (191) **W R**
FEMALE; PAIN; General; ovaries (K731, G623) (170) **R**
FEMALE; PAIN; stitching; ovaries (K742, G630) (52) **R**

COUGH; AIR; cold; sensation of cold air in throat (1) **R N**
COUGH; SPICES, condiments, highly seasoned food agg. (K790, G672) (4) **R**

CHEST; PAIN; stitching (K863, G728) (349) **R**
CHEST; PAIN; stitching; inspiration; amel. (2) **R**
CHEST; SWELLING; Mammae; menses; before and during (1) **W N**

BACK; PAIN; General; bending; agg.; forward (K895, G753) (5) **R**

EXTREMITIES; ERUPTIONS; Fingers (K996, G832) (78) **R**
EXTREMITIES; INJURIES; Hand (1) **W N**

EXTREMITIES; INJURIES; Fingers (28) W R
EXTREMITIES; PERSPIRATION; Foot (K1183, G979) (156) W
EXTREMITIES; PERSPIRATION; Foot; offensive (K1183, G979) (58) W
EXTREMITIES; PERSPIRATION; Foot; offensive; cheese,
    Gouda cheese (1) W N
EXTREMITIES; PERSPIRATION; Foot; warm (K1184, G979) (2) W
EXTREMITY PAIN; UPPER LIMBS; Shoulder (K1051, G875) (271) W

SLEEP; SLEEPINESS (K1248, SIII-82, G1030) (575) W R
SLEEP; SLEEPINESS; daytime (61) W R
SLEEP; SLEEPINESS; heaviness, with (SIII-109) (12) W R
SLEEP; SLEEPINESS; sitting, while (K1251, SIII-119, G1032) (79) W R
SLEEP; SLEEPLESSNESS; evening; bed, after going to (K1252, SIII-132, G1033)
    (16) W R
SLEEP; SLEEPLESSNESS; weariness; in spite of weariness (SIII-184) (31) W
SLEEP; UNREFRESHING (K1254, SIII-186, G1035) (240) W R
SLEEP; WAKING; urinate, with desire to (SIII-214) (16) R

CHILL; NIGHT; bed, in; agg. (K1261, G1041) (20) W

PERSPIRATION; ODOR; offensive; cheese, like (2) W

SKIN; ITCHING (K1327, G1094) (334) R

GENERALITIES; FOOD and drinks; cold; drinks, water; desires (K484, SII-233,
G414) (156) W R
GENERALITIES; FOOD and drinks; sweets; desires
    (K486, SII-274, G415) (107) W R
GENERALITIES; FOOD and drinks; sweets; desires; soft, and (1) W R N
GENERALITIES; FOOD and drinks; tea; desires
    (K486, SII-276, G415) (19) W R
GENERALITIES; HEAVINESS; internally; lead, as of (2) W
GENERALITIES; INJURIES, blows, falls and bruises
    (K1368, SII-323, G1129) (220) W R
GENERALITIES, PAIN; pressing; internally (K1382, SII-438, G1140) (201) W R
GENERALITIES; PAIN; wandering (K1389, SII-475, G1146) (162) W
GENERALITIES; SIDE; right (K1400, SII-590, G1155) (227) W R
GENERALITIES; SUDDEN manifestations (SII-616) (59) W R
GENERALITIES; WEAKNESS, enervation, exhaustion, prostration, infirmity;
alternating with; activity (5) W

GENERALITIES; WEARINESS; tendency (K1421, SII-745, G1170) (252) **W** **R**
GENERALITIES; WEARINESS; tendency; evening; agg.
    (K1421, SII-747, G1171) (16) **W** **R**
GENERALITIES; WEARINESS; tendency; sudden (1) **R** **N**
GENERALITIES; WOUNDS; cuts (K1422, SII-768, G1172) (26) **R**

Comment:
We, as the authors, gave it a lot of thought as to whether or not it would be a good idea to differentiate between the two different types of 'Vitis' according to nomenclature, with white here and red there - ie whether to also differentiate between them in the repertory using different rubric abbreviations for each - e.g. vitis-w. and vitis-r, or vitis-fol. (Folia - for the leaves) and vitis-fr. (Fructibus - for the fruit).

We then, however, decided not to do this, even though with some effort, logistically, it would definitely have been feasible. Consequently for the time being it will be up to the readers, and those who prescribe Vitis, to see if individual symptoms belong to the one or the other, by referring to the preceding list or in the proving journals.

Vitis vinifera in practice –
a red wine grape case study [J.W.]

Johanna, 42 years old, secretary/student (social worker)
Anaemia, debility, chronic headaches

Appearance:
Johanna always wears clothes that blend well together, earthy colours, preferably brown or dark-red.
She has somewhat droopy upper eyelids (ptosis).

"I have come about my anaemia. I feel so worn out, very tired and my resistance is very low."
She has been like this for 2 years, getting worse all the time. Anaemia was diagnosed six months ago.
"I have had psoriasis since I was 17, particularly on the elbows, knees and ankles. My skin flares up when I am tense and under stress. Holidays, the sun and seaside have a distinctly beneficial effect on my skin."

Clinical observations:
The skin eruptions are very symmetrical; identical patches of psoriasis are visible on both sides of the extremities.

"The symmetrical aspect fits me well. I like harmony and order. That applies to my clothes as well as at home.
Periods are heavy, my cycle has been up and down over the last months. The blood is always dark, and lots of clots. I am very thin-skinned before my period, cry at the slightest thing. I prefer to keep to myself at this time. Everyone wants something from me, but at this time I don't want anything from anyone."

110

"I gave up my job as a secretary five years ago. At the moment I am halfway through my studies. As a result of this I have also given up my (financial) independence from my husband. Since then everything causes pressure and tension in my life.

You know, I am very organised and since I have been studying I sometimes have to leave things until later because I just can't get around to them. The course is not so easy for me, I am the oldest and really have to make an effort to take everything in."

Observation:
She has to laugh all the time when she is talking, even when it's about serious things:

"I feel like I have to give 150% to everything. And then if, in addition to that, I feel I'm being assessed it is absolutely horrible for me. Since I started studying this obviously creates exceptional pressure for me. And when I'm under pressure, that is the time when I often have these headaches. My head feels as if it is in a vice.

My husband is not very good about boundaries. We frequently have problems about who is responsible for what. It is a constant strain, but it doesn't seem to bother him much. I like to be in a harmonious environment and don't like arguing."

Childhood/Biography:
"My parents had a terrible marriage. Father was a miner. He was an alcoholic and there was also a lot of violence at home. He used to beat my mother.

It was my job to even things out, to be a facilitator. They divorced when I was sixteen. My sister and I stayed with my mother. I went to my father's funeral, not having had any contact with him beforehand. My mother was tough, she was always a fighter, also fighting for a better world. She usually suppressed her own needs. And she was very bitter. She usually delegated things and passed them on to me (I was the oldest). She also liked to hand over responsibility to me. We were never allowed to enjoy life. We weren't allowed any pleasure. And so I left my mother when I was young and have tried to stand on my own two feet and earn my own money (from 17 years old)."

Fears:
"Of arguing, which results in you losing someone.
Darkness - being alone
Heights, I can't look down from high up."

"I never wanted to have children, because of my awful childhood. I'm sad about that now, as time has passed.

I'm a good listener. It sometimes wears me out, because I pick up other people's signals and feel responsible for the person opposite me most of the time. I can tell

111

what's going on, on a deeper level and that often causes a dilemma for me. And that always happened to me with my mother. I felt responsible for her happiness."

"I had a slipped disc in the autumn of 1994. Since then I have back pain frequently."

Desires
Food: "Sweets, potatoes, meat. I enjoy my food generally. That's how I reward myself, particularly with sweets. I am a hedonist.
Drinks: Tea, red wine."

Aversion
"Muscles and other marine creatures, fish, milk."

Temperature
"My feet get cold quickly.
I am having night sweats frequently at the moment."

Digestion
"I am constipated most of the time and have to really strain for any success."

Dreams
"One dream comes to mind straight away. Something I want to tell you ... I don't have a driver's licence and don't know how to drive. I never liked the idea of driving because you have to do so many things at once.
Well, in the dream I can drive all of a sudden. I'm driving around all over the place, but then woke up bathed in sweat."

Analysis and prescription
At the time of the first consultation with this patient I didn't as yet have a good picture of Vitis vinifera. The repertory rubrics had also yet to be compiled.
A lot of the themes in this case reminded me of Sepia (no resistance to illnesses, connection with the sea (aversion to fish, psoriasis > by the seaside), difficult relationship with one's father, perfectionism, difficulty with boundaries, weeping before menses etc.)
There were also some Magnesium themes (child with divorced parents, can't argue, fear of losing someone, obsessed with harmony).
But I couldn't bring myself to prescribe either Sepia or on the connection with the Magnesium's.
It was the strong polarity between the themes of perfection, harmony and symmetry (just like the way the vines are cultivated and grown) and the 'hedonist' who has to reward herself, which got me thinking of the red wine proving initially.

The likewise similar problem with boundaries, that can be found in Sepia, appeared as a curative symptom for a number of Vitis provers. They were more able to define their boundaries and saw things from a more easy-going perspective. Of all the provers, prover 12 expressed this the most clearly in her journal:

"There is always a lot of things to do in my family and work life. On the one hand I like these activities, on the other hand I become overwhelmed by a kind of fear of excessive demands being put upon me. Fear that I won't be able to manage to have things under control. Then I usually fall into a certain kind of depression, which is not visible to others. Thanks to the proving none of this has occurred this year and everything has been fine! I was a lot more relaxed about things, things were going well."

The dream about driving provided me with a further, decisive indication to prescribe Vitis vinifera. She is anxious when driving a car, what happens when several things have to be done simultaneously (fear of loss of control?).

Provers were out and about a lot in cars during both the white and red wine proving (often very dangerously!). For example, prover 10 dreamt: "When we come to drive away we notice that our front wheels have been dismantled and the suspension had been damaged. My husband steps into action and gets the farmer's son to help him. I start to become concerned about whether we can get down to the bottom of the hillside in the van in one piece." *(The patient can't look down from above!!). The oppressive headaches were also an indication for Vitis. She had the sensation as if her head was in a vice (in wine production the grapes are often squashed in an old wooden press under enormous pressure!)*

Prescription: Vitis vinifera 30c (Red Spätburgunder)

1st follow up, 6 weeks later

"Normally I can hardly ever remember my dreams in great detail. But this time I had some really peculiar dreams.
What is more I was flipping out and getting furious over every little thing, in a way I've never done before."

Dream: "I was holding my mother in my arms like you do with a small child, being very protective. My father kept going past (in a threatening way). I kept trying to maintain eye contact with him. I was thinking I'm not going to be able to keep this up for long, and then I woke."

"I was really furious on a lot of occasions. Judging by the extent of the anger that surfaced, it must have been from long ago. I also wanted to hit out, to just beat up anyone who got in my way."

Dream: "My husband has drowned. I wanted to help him but I didn't get there in time." *(Johanna narrated this dream in a very matter-of-fact way, and somehow with the message, well I was just too late).*

Dream: "Just a bit of a dream: A bomb has exploded (atom bomb)."

"On the whole I'm more energetic. For the first time in my life I have experienced how it is to be on the other side. For the first time in my life I was able to understand how it is for the person opposite me (my father who was always threatening)."

"Headaches have reduced considerably, only bad once when my mother came to visit. I had to protect my mother all my life. When I am with her I feel like a fish out of water."

Analysis/Strategy
Her energy has clearly improved, her headaches are less frequent. She is more in touch with her life purpose and can see how it is to be on 'the other side' for the first time in her life. All of this indicates a good start to treatment.
Action: No remedy, wait.

Phone call between consultation (8 weeks after first dose of 30c), there has been a distinct decrease in energy.
Prescription: Vitis vinifera 200c

2nd follow up, 4 weeks later (after 200c)

"Once again I had amazing dreams. I was doing things that I am not usually able to. For example. I was standing on a stage in my dream and singing in the choir (I can't sing at all!!).
This time my dreams were only about me.
I feel like I'm more in touch with myself. My energy level has increased considerably, compared with before my treatment. My cycle is still shorter (every 21 days). Still bleeding heavily but the period is over quicker. My skin is up and down (psoriasis), I can't see any improvement there.
I just feel like I've got more energy.
I still tend to get annoyed quicker. I still feel like I could hit out. It feels so good to get it out."

114

Dream: "I was riding right through the city. It was a wonderful feeling to be riding, though I don't actually know how to!!). When I arrived at my destination I realised that I didn't know what I was meant to do with the horse. It was a large, dark horse."

Analysis/Strategy
The fact that Johanna is riding right through the city and feels wonderful doing it gives us reason to believe that there is hope for continued liberation of her inner strength.
She was very surprised initially and also scared, but now she really seems to benefit from being able to get in touch with her 'vibrancy' (libido).

Action: Wait, no prescription.

3rd follow up, 10 weeks after Vitis 200c

"It was less of a roller coaster."

"For the first time in my life I have noticed that I have sexual needs. It really is a completely new feeling for me. My husband always had a healthy sexual appetite but I didn't. When I got married I thought that was just how things were. I had a few one-night stands before I met my husband but only really for contact. I always felt ashamed when it came to sex. When I was about 10 years old my father started to abuse me.
I am becoming aware that during that time I completely suppressed something."

"I have had no headaches whatsoever since the last dose of the remedy. I am absolutely positive that my headaches were connected with the suppressed sexuality. The only thing that I have still been experiencing recently is a humming in my head when I'm angry."

"What really annoys me at the moment is my husband's depressive side. I use up so much of my energy trying to drag him out of it."

"During the last few weeks I had several dreams related to sex, and once it had something to do with rape."
Dream: "My friend had been raped by her boyfriend. In the dream I asked her how come she didn't put up a fight? She replied that that's just how it is and she just let it happen. Then her boyfriend came out of the room and I perceived it as a threat; that he could do the same thing to me. And then I woke up."

Menses
Continues to occur every 21 days, with heavy bleeding but not lasting as long.

Sleep
Noticeably more restful.

Analysis/strategy
I was certainly thrilled. There have been huge changes in the patient - as indicated by the aforementioned 'horse dream'. During treatment I never questioned her about her sexuality directly. She has 'worked out' all these things on her own, bit by bit. She also appears to be working through the abuse. So far everything is happening on a level that she and those around her can handle.

The patient describes her husband as depressive and rigid, which causes me some concern for their further development together.

Action: No remedy. Wait.

There was some turbulence over the next six months, particularly on the physical level. First of all her blood pressure escalated. She spoke about 'feeling like a pressure cooker' and feeling under tremendous pressure.
She decided to act on her feelings and attended a 'Tao and Sexuality' seminar. Her marriage was really being put to the test, but they managed for it not to come to separation, and are still together (3 year observation period). Their arguments are far more constructive. There is give and take.

The next crisis came when her blood sugar went off the rails. She then also confessed that for years she would always have an additional particular portion of sweets in the evening to get her to sleep. 'It's part of my ritual before I go to sleep to have something sweet.' The principle of gratification (as in the initial consultation) just isn't working any more. This all became apparent when a skin eruption, causing soreness under both breasts, wouldn't heal. Johanna then went on a sugar-free diet and within a short period of time lost 4 kilos.

During this period she had 2 doses of Vitis vinifera 1m.

During this time I viewed the crises that she was experiencing on the physical level with great discernment and wasn't always sure that Vitis was still the right remedy for her.
However, over a period of time (3 year observation period) both the blood pressure and the blood sugar stabilised completely without the intervention of orthodox medication. Actually by losing weight she has also acquired a new physical appearance and an attractiveness, which she is very happy about.

116

The tendency to 'lose it' when she's taken for granted is something she has held onto. This is then reflected again in a later dream, which has to do with her place in the family (system).

"The dream takes place in my parent's kitchen. The table has been set for four. All the seats were taken, however. Someone from our neighbourhood was sitting in my place. This person looked like my mother and yet also like my father's sister. I was incredibly angry that she'd taken my place. I took her plate away but she didn't move. I then shouted at her, like I have never done in my whole life."

Analysis / strategy

Vitis vinifera was a wonderful remedy for this patient for 3 years. She resolved and sorted out a lot of things in her life. She no longer has anaemia or headaches. She managed to break out from the repression and to live a fuller life, more in touch with her emotions. The same kind of story we often hear after Sepia, Carcinosin or the Magnesium salts.

Her energy and vitality are back in a way that she has not known for a long time, or possibly has never experienced before. The largest benefit however has come through her dreams. Most of the time they indicated that changes were imminent.

As so often happens when a remedy has a profound effect on us, it is the dreams that guide us and when we listen to their message and let them take us by the hand they lead us gently a little closer to our true self.

Ideas about Vitis

Search for something to hold on to, restraint & over-indulgence [P.K.]

As already mentioned, it was the signatures in the provers' dreams that pointed the way for us in comprehending the remedy: Vitis on the dream stage, the stage director disguised in the role of the actor, so to speak - a fact that is witnessed time and again in provings! These two dreams, by the same prover, call the remedy by it's name and, at the same time, pick something out as a central theme, which could be the basic idea behind Vitis vinifera: the search for **something to hold on to.**

Night: I dream that I am driving (a female friend was in the passenger seat). I am driving particularly dangerously (but not responding to it) and when we come to a bend the car skids across the road. We are thrown from the car and plunge down an incline. My friend grabs hold of me and I am able to reduce our speed by repeatedly clinging to shrubs and by doing this we come away unscathed. (6m/10 [last day of the proving])

Dream: My mother is driving the car and has to brake hard suddenly. I'm flung out of the car and am thrown quite a distance: beneath me are vines with trellises running parallel and as I'm flying through the air I wonder how my fall is going to be. I try to land causing as little damage as possible, i.e. I plunge into the vines and brake with my left hand. As I land I notice that I have hardly any injuries, except for a cut on the left hand. They take me to the hospital, my mother is driving too slowly, and very badly. My father is sitting in the back, pretty annoyed with her and wants to take over the driving. (6m/19P)

118

In the first dream, in which the friend is grabbing hold of the dreamer, and the dreamer clinging to the shrubs by the side of the road, both individuals are experiencing how it is trying to save themselves. In the second dream it is the vine trellises running 'in parallel lines' (in the follow-up following the proving he said he meant wire trellis) that helped him to slow down - even if it did injure him.

Vitis vinifera is a creeper and twiner (see the chapter entitled 'Vitis vinifera the plant') as are many of the plants in our materia medica, amongst others Humulus lupulus, hops! - A selection of these plants are mentioned in Table 2:

creepers in homoeopathy

actin.	actinidia chinensis
bani-c.	banisteriopsis caapi
bry.	bryonia cretica (- dioica)
bry-a.	bryonia alba
calam.	calamus aromaticus (acorus calamus)
cocc.	cocculus indicus
coloc.	colocynthis
cuc-p.	cucurbita pepo
cund.	cundurango
cur.	curare
cusc.	cuscuta europaea
dulc.	dulcamara
elat.	elaterium officinarum
gels.	gelsemium sempervirens
hed.	hedera helix
ign.	ignatia amara
luf-op.	luffa operculata
lup.	lupulus humulus
lupin.	lupulinum
mom-b.	momordica balsamica
passi.	passiflora incarnata
phase.	phaseolus nanus
phase-vg.	phaseolus vulgaris
pip-n.	piper nigrum
pis-s.	pisum sativum
rhus-r.	rhus radicans
sars.	sarsaparilla officinalis
vitis	vitis vinifera

Table 2

We also notice the connection between the 'holding on' and the symptoms of dizziness observed by our provers. Cocculus Indicus also appears in this list of climbing plants.

Our hands are the parts of our bodies we use predominantly to get a grip on life. It seems significant that during both of our Vitis provings the theme of injuries to hands and fingers came up frequently. In the Austrian white wine proving mainly in dreams, whereas a real life experience for Jürgen Weiland in the red wine proving.

It seems plausible to project these impressive, above mentioned dream images internally, i.e. the external holding onto an object: Holding on to something externally turns into holding onto something internally.

The signature of the vine - except in southern regions, where vines grow more freely - has characteristics of discipline and 'domestication', as a consequence of interactions with civilised man: Rank and file cultivation, - tied up high (in German wine language 'High Culture') tied loosely[20] , strung up, cut back rigourously, the wild shoots cut out, in order to force the plant to produce maximum yield. In wine vocabulary the word training[21] (G: Erziehung) is used regarding this. The image of a crooked, crippled, knotted, deformed, many-eyed piece of woody vine clearly illustrates this[22] . The soil for wine has to be barren, not rich, and without too much humus. In addition, high-culture grapevines are artificially kept under stress, in order to increase competition for nutrients between the individual plants. This is done to improve the quality of the grapes: the fewer the grapes, the greater the pleasure to come!

But the 'wildness' in wine is still present. In our (wine) culture it is in the form of the 'base vine'. This became necessary as a result of attack by root-

---

20 According to Genaust the etymological meaning of 'Vitis' (as also the willow) originates from the Indo-Germanic root 'ueit' which means something along the lines of 'to bend', 'to twine'.

21 'Consideration has to be given in the first year already, as to which type of training is to be chosen.' (Wunderer)

22 In the animal kingdom it is the dog (Lac caninum) which comes closest in this domestication of the formerly untamed - and also in its imprisonment in the history of human evolution.

inhabiting phylloxera in these latitudes since the 19th century. And so it is that 'wild' sap streams upwards into these highly cultivated 'high class' specialised plants, which are prone to disease.

Consequently wine possesses, as was mentioned in the introduction, almost human characteristics. In historical terms regarding wine one speaks of an increased 'individualisation' and 'personality' of wine ('One drinks the winegrower'). The characteristics of various wines are given human traits in an almost rapturous fashion: delicate, open-minded, animated, playful, approachable, congenial, as well as a 'Dining Companion'. In 'Talking to Vines' Peter Gutting writes about a visit to a Demeter vineyard (In the periodical 'Schrot & Korn' 10/2002), and refers to an 'attentive dialogue between soil and vine'. Another quote, this time by winegrower Hartmut Heintz: 'In a good wine you can taste the landscape and the people living in it ...'

A special characteristic of this type of 'high cultivation' is a heightened sense of (social) responsibility. Early clinical experiences with Vitis vinifera (J.W., see the chapter with the Vitis case) depict Vitis patients as possessing a high degree of responsibility (similar to Aurum and Carcinosin). However, Vitis seems to resemble Staphisagria more in this manner, with it's tendency to go though life putting aside it's own needs - more so than we would expect from Aurum.

Human/soldier-like qualities have been more or less imposed upon the vine, or to be precise, the plant, has allowed this be imposed upon it. It holds back and even sacrifices it's own wildness in order to enable high cultivation. Under these aspects of the vine, those who take the signature seriously may find the Vitis symptoms more comprehensible and meaningful: The striking, colourful, manifold animal dreams being the part in us which is unleashed. Prover 13m's impulsive outbursts - both psychologically as well as in flatulence! - as also the bursting forth of 'wild instinctual energy' of animalistic nature, which has hitherto been kept under reins with great difficulty.

Someone who has lost his/her inner hold on life, who walks through life 'dizzily', may instead look for and find it externally in drugs (ie in wine). And the person who fails to meet external demands of discipline, may switch to addictive behaviour and may become an alcoholic. Grapevines, however, do not always grow in rank and file in our vineyards. In an old illustration of a playful configuration of a grapevine[23], this plant grows brazenly through a gap in an adjoining tree - in contrast

---

23 ' From various features and characteristics of the grape vine': Woodcutting from

to the military, almost conciliatory picture, giving an indication of some further potential of the Vitis plant, which still also needs to be considered from a homeopathic viewpoint:

In his Dionysiaca[24], Nonnus describes the grape vine (and it's dependence on other plants) in the richest of terms:

> '..and others sparkled altogether
> Blackish blue like tar, and,
> intoxicated the olive trees close by and their
> shimmering fruits with their entwined grapevines.

We obviously can't just simplify the signature as being a suppression of impulses as in that of a soldier. First and foremost we cannot look at our Vitis picture from this one angle only. Are we therefore saying that we have hitherto forgotten about Dionysus, about the aphrodisiacal aspects of wine consumption (Rätsch)? What we have been calling 'wild', ought to be described in new terms, taking into account the signature-like lavish growth of the grape vine's tendrils. In his book on botanical medicines, Pelikan describes Vitis in quite a flowery fashion: ' ... arbitrary roaming, playfully winding and gripping, horizontally broadening like hands made of leaves, lavishly swelling, weighty, hanging grapes ... playful fantasy'. It is these characteristics, that are neither suppressed nor sublimated, that also need to be considered from a homeopathic perspective!

We assume, or, to be precise, we are convinced that, in order to develop a deeper understanding of Vitis as a homeopathic remedy, it is necessary not to engage in over-simplistic mono-causal psychological constructs, which implies that a (hitherto) misunderstood dichotomy can stand side by side.

---

the 14th century by von P. Creszenzi, taken from '12 Books about the Usefulness of Farming'
24 Nonnus' Dionysiaca 12 (p. 292 in German version) by Rätsch, Healing Herbs in Classical Antiquity, in Egypt, Greece and Rome

Vitis - Alcoholus - Vinum ?
What does the Vine know about the Wine? [P.K.]

Can the effect of a remedy be explained by its components? To our knowledge this has yet to be answered, although Jan Scholten for instance provides us at least with some answers in his system using the Periodic Table. In my view, the effect of a homeopathic remedy is NOT wholly deducible from the knowledge of the individual components - just as a human being cannot be explained by the sum of the combined functions of his/her organs. Here we clearly come up against the philosophical question to do with the 'nature', 'essence' (Vithoulkas), 'soul' of a remedy.

So: 'Vinum' is NOT equal to 'Vitis' plus 'Alcoholus'! But: In Vinum, there would have to be some evidence of Alcoholus and Vitis symptoms. There would have to be at least a trace that can be followed up. Vitis is the only one of these three substances to have been proved. In the literature Vinum can at most only be found as an antidote, and Alcoholus symptoms derive from experiments with substantial dosages, as well as symptoms of poisoning and alcoholism. Consequently, due to the absence of systematic foundations, this possible search for clues appears hopeless from the start.

Yet it seems so much more tempting - and this has also happened to us repeatedly after the uncovering of the proved remedy - to use the facts we know about wine and its effects as the basis for individual symptoms, in the sense of an 'aha, I see, experience', - e.g. with the dizziness- or headache-symptoms, or with the dreams full of animals (see later in the text), which remind us of the delirium experienced in alcohol withdrawal. We know from clinical experience that these patients have frightening delusions and images of animals ('elementary hallucinations'), e.g. beetles, rats, black cats or bears. With our knowledge from the outcome of the Vitis proving, it seems absolutely necessary to ask the question whether these images of animals also occurred amongst the withdrawal symptoms of notorious spirit or beer drinkers, or was it only with wine-drinkers that they occurred. This could be an indication that in this case - in the non-potentised toxic sphere! - genuine Vitis symptoms accompany such a delirium. Certainly chronic alcoholics generally consume a variety of alcoholic drinks, and mix their drinks, so this question will have to remain unanswered. Also, the theme of looking for something to hold on to brings to mind the unsteady drinker (of wine?) who is looking for something to 'hold onto', not only in the sense in which it is being conveyed, but often also in the actual sense, e.g. a lamppost.

Without the grape vine and its fruits, the grapes, there would be no wine (and as a result of that some things in this world would be somewhat different?!), but there would most certainly be other intoxicating alcoholic drinks if it were not for Vitis vinifera. Following our Vitis presentation at the World Congress in Sibiu, a question was asked from the audience (Friedrich Dellmour), probably also as an attempt to explain the reference to alcohol in our Vitis symptoms: Does the plant Vitis 'know' of its future use as wine, in the same way as Sepia 'knows' of the sea? Perhaps there is a 'field' that links up information about 'grape vine' and 'wine' in several directions, possibly even about the experiences and the information gathered by the individual remedy prover. Dellmour asks the (hitherto unanswered) question, whether different proving symptoms would be observed with people who had never been in contact with wine as opposed to people who have 'stored' the information on 'wine' with its many associations. My reply (P.K.'s, in writing at the time) pointed out that an (already complicated) matter was in danger of becoming even more complicated: For is not everything we have experienced in life 'linked up'?

Wouldn't then some people proving a metallic element for instance, then also be able to produce proving symptoms of all sorts of alloys and their applications, as known to them? From my point of view it is already complex enough, with all the 'anecdotes' that such a substance brings along with it, that are incorporated into it (e.g. the information regarding the 'sea' in Sepia[25])...

For me it is more probable that the substances themselves bring the knowledge of their purpose and utilisation of them, in the sense that e.g. Vitis, for example, contains the 'potential' to be particularly suitable for the making of an intoxicating drink (wine). Perhaps both views are also not exclusive of one another.

We know from ancient sources that unfermented grape juice (uncultivated wine) was consumed during Dionysian rituals. Is it, therefore, possible that there is an intoxicating Vitis component beyond the alcoholic content in wine?

---

25 Regarding the phenomena being discussed here, there is a possible simple explanation relating to Vitis in particular: In his book 'Healing Plants' Pelikan mentions that the yeast spores on the grape, which contribute to the fermentation process, sit on the berry's skin: 'What is needed for the fermentation process is already there and waiting'.

Animals and Vitis [P.K.]

We have already attempted to explain Vitis' 'Noah's Ark', our above mentioned provers' animal dreams, on the basis of the delirium experienced during alcohol-withdrawal. This brings to mind yet another idea which refers to mythology:

The 'shamanic' god Dionysus also has animal spirits as helpers and can take on the identity of animals (Rätsch): panther, lynx, lion, tiger, dolphin, snake, bull, ram. We have already mentioned that animal images in our dreams may represent the part in us that remains 'untamed' [26]. The fact that Vitis (wine) is able to release these qualities, which are often covered up, is not only demonstrated by the experience of grape juice in it's 'mother tincture' form, but also by our proving.

What exactly is a badger doing in prover 1f's Vitis dream? I obtained the following information and to some extent signature-like associations from a participant in one of my (P.K.) lectures, who had studied badgers for some time: Badgers like to dig their tunnels in soil where vines grow. Furthermore, amongst various fruits the badgers eat, they are particularly partial to grapes.

Badgers are highly refined in the manner by which they deposit their droppings - referred to as the 'badger's loo'. On the other hand, the badger is regarded as a grumpy, bad tempered animal, which can also behave extremely aggressively ...

Vitis Affinity with Beer or Wine Drinkers [P.K.]

It was an interesting question for us as to whether a proving substance, which plays such a major part in our everyday lives as a secondary product (in the

---

26 Aeppli on this subject : Animal symbols are able to express the course of our actions, the type and strength of the orientation of our desires through the allegory of their nature. The animal has become a symbol for the tamed and untamed in us, and for the most simple and seemingly incomprehensible in our nature. In animal analogy we recognise that which hurries through the air of our thoughts, that which walks on the strong earth of our day, that which dwells in the forest of our unconscious or that which lives in the dark oceans of our depths from long ago as the autonomous inner life.

form of wine) can cause (more or less powerful) symptoms with people who have a particular affinity with this beverage - either as 'wine drinkers' or those who totally reject it. As we are familiar with the polarisation of beer or wine drinkers, we have attempted to include these aspects in the formulation of our question.

To this end we have compiled a table to illustrate our provers' affinity for wine/beer on a scale of -3 (total rejection), 0 (indifference) to +3 (strong craving). A simple totalling up of the numbers on table 3 gives us the following representation:

	Wine	Beer
7 "best responders"	+6	+2
8 other provers	+11	+12

Table 3

Comments: It has become apparent that those provers who reacted well to Vitis (our sensitive provers) tended not to be partial to wine in their drinking habits. Prover 1 (1f) who provided us with so many and such distinct Vitis symptoms, doesn't even like wine. Whether this has something to do with the male provers being represented more in the 'remaining provers' group and therefore increasing the affinity to wine to +11? The contrast becomes even more apparent with cravings for beer.

Disregarding the possibility of statistical distortions due to the male/female ratio, one could conclude (possibly somewhat generalised) that, with female provers who in everyday life don't demonstrate such a distinct affinity to wine (through direct contact with a proving substance), the interactions with the proving substance Vitis are noticeably stronger. This issue would need to be researched further.

Regulation of heat and cold
(Snow)-white & (Blood)-red [J.W.]

We saw many overlaps in the results of the provings of both varieties of grapes, which spurred us on to go ahead with a joint publication. Thankfully there were also significant differences in how the provers reacted to the individual provings. These could perhaps be what will tip the scales in favour of the one or

126

other type when prescribing Vitis in the future.

We observed a significant and distinctive lack of vital heat in the 'white provers' in direct comparison to the 'red provers' who often felt a pleasant feeling of warmth. What aspects might have caused that?

The mother tincture for the white wine proving was extracted in spring from fresh leaves. They would have absorbed fewer hours of sunshine than the red grapes, which were gathered in autumn and formed the basis for the red wine proving. Certainly the pigment of the blood-red grape, compared to the light, cooler colour of the white grape suggests a difference in the regulation of heat observed in the two remedies.

Injuries, accidents and bites [J.W.]

Results from the proving depict a correspondence in the type and frequency of accidents and injuries, or mutilations. Whereas the 'white provers' experienced accidents and injuries in their dreams (the badger biting the hand), for the 'red provers' the injuries were more real (cut from a bread knife). In general the red wine proving left the provers with a 'deeper penetrating impression'.

One possible explanation for these different phenomena between white and red could have to do with the different signatures of the two different types of grape: as a result of it's high anthocyanin and tannic acid content the red grape demonstrates a positively aggressive side, compared to that of the white grape.

This is also reflected in the many combined skin symptoms from both Vitis provings. In direct comparison, the red wine provers demonstrated more invasive lesions on the skin and mucous membranes than the white wine provers.

Clinical footnotes : Fungal infections and miscarriage [P.K.]

The fact that that there is an evidently undeniable affinity between Vitis and fungal organisms, as seen by the signature of the plant Vitis - both the possible effect of pest infestation as also the would-be fermentation process on the berry's skin as a result of yeast spores - suggests exploration into a clinical interconnection regarding fungal affections in humans. Apart from prover 1f's foot sweat that smelt like cheese (possibly as a predisposition to fungal infections) and prover 13m's offensive flatulence, in addition to the many symptoms affecting the mucous membranes in various provers - Candida?! - we do not have any indications to support this from the proving symptoms. There is a noticeable absence of additional skin and/or genital symptoms that would be needed to indicate this. Pryce and Langcake describe a fungicidal substance as being an element of the vine tendril.

From conversations with Jürgen Weiland, shaped by all of the authors' deep personal experiences, we feel it is permissible to make a connection between Vitis and the theme of miscarriage and threatening miscarriage: Holding on to a child that does not want (or is not allowed) to 'go'. On the subject of the signature of the vine we also see how, as a result of having roots that penetrate deep into the ground, it has the ability to survive, no matter what. And what about the walking stick made from vine which, once it has been positioned in the earth and left there for a long time, establishes roots!

Possible connections with other remedies [P.K. & J.W.]

Cocculus has already been mentioned as a collateral remedy regarding it's vertigo - as also **Lycopodium**: See prover 13m's proving symptoms for more on this. What is particularly noticeable is the amount of times that **Magnesiums** come up in the rubrics that we have added Vitis to. **Staphisagria** stands out amongst other things for its mucous membrane symptoms that are similar to Vitis; the connection with injuries and it's tendency to suppress anger.

Sepia worked very well as antidote for Prover 10f (for toothache). The relationship to Sepia and the Magnesiums was evident from the earlier mentioned case history. (q.v.) [J.W.]

Acknowledgements

Austrian proving

Our thanks for the actualization of this contribution into the homeopathic Materia Medica go firstly to the provers, without whose contribution, diligence and talent for self-observation Vitis would have certainly remained undeveloped to this present day.

Thanks to Robert Müntz, the friendly, reliable, encouraging pharmacist at Salvathor Pharmacy in Eisenstadt (www.remedia.at) for choosing and producing the proving remedy.

All the people who directly or indirectly played a role at the Vitis seminar in January 2002 in Eisenstadt:

Helmut Gangl, Graduate Engineer and Institute Manager at the Austrian Federal Office for Viticulture in Eisenstadt,
Dr Walter Flak, Director of the above mentioned Federal Office,
Christian Kurz, ND and Doctor of physics, for his suggestions, both relating to homeopathy and also as a wine connoisseur - and particularly for his preface on our 'Vitis'.
Councillor Norbert Springschütz from the Prince of Esterházy's Foundation at Castle Eisenstadt for letting us sample a wonderful Green Veltliner at the end of the seminar and for letting us use the premises of the Esterházy restaurant,

... Miriam Wiegele from Weiden bei Rechnitz in southern Burgenland who provided us with references about Vitis regarding botany, cultural history and the art of healing,

... Dr Rosmarie Mayr, Consultant Psychiatrist from Salzburg, for valuable information about withdrawal symptoms from alcohol,

... Eda Camus for conscientiously typing up the hand-written proving journals into the computer,

... the couple, Johanna Rattner-Eggl and Gerhard Rattner from 'Kräuterwirt' in Prein an der Rax, who made their house and their culinary art available to us so that we could conduct our proving undisturbed from 26th to 28th July 2002...

... Father Alois Schwarztischer from the Apostolatshaus der Pallottiner in Salzburg, where we hatched our combined version of Vitis, who empathetically provided us with literature on 'Wine and the Bible' ...

... Jörg Wichmann, Fagus Verlag, Rösrath, for taking on Vitis in his series of publications, and also for his words of encouragement and inspiration ...

German Proving

My thanks first of all to the provers and their supervisors, for their willingness and their courage for having taken part in this double blind study. I would also like to pay particular thanks to the provers for their physical commitment in physical terms. The 'red wine' bequeathed small and somewhat larger injuries (refer to accidents). However after seeking reassurance from the 'injured parties' at the end of the proving these produced a valuable experience on a different level, causing no-one to regret the proving.

I would also like to thank my colleagues

Dr. Gisela Nordhorn-Richter, for the advice relating to biology/botany. She encouraged me to use the 'ripe' grape.

Ulrike Wölbert, my clinic assistant at the time, who supported me tremendously during the grape harvest and the processing of the mother tincture.

The pharmacist Sven Göbel, in whose Löwen Pharmacy in Meckenheim we carried out the potentisation from the 3c trituration.

My friend and colleague Jörg Wichmann for his commitment (see above).

Christoph Bäcker, the winegrower from the Ahr (www.weingutbaecker.de) from whose vineyard the mother tincture originates. His ecologically cultivated wine is really a very special vintage.

Also thanks to my wife Sabine, who accompanied this proving with patience and loving support.

130

Literature and other Vitis sources

Aeppli, E.: Der Traum und seine Bedeutung. (The dream and it's Interpretation) Knaur, München 1984.

Bastian, H. (Hrsg.): Ullstein Lexikon der Pflanzenwelt. (Encyclopaedia of the Plant World) Verlag Ullstein, Frankfurt – Berlin - Wien 1973.

Bauer, W.;Dümotz,I.; Golowin S.: Lexikon der Symbole, (Encyclopaedia of Symbols) Fourier Verlag Wiesbaden, 16. Aufl. 1996.

Dominé, A.: Wein. (Wine) Könemann, Köln 2000. Translated edition 2001.

Euripides: Die Backchen. (The Bacchants) Wiesbaden-Berlin. Vollmer Verlag.

Genaust, H.: Etymologisches Wörterbuch der botanischen Pflanzennamen, 3. Aufl. (Etymological Dictionary of Botanical Plant Names, 3rd edition) Birkhäuser, Basel – Bosoton – Berlin, 1996.

Hahnemann, S.: Organon der Heilkunst, Ausgabe 6B, (Organon of Medicine, edition 6B) Kurt Hochstetter, Haug-Verlag.

Jung, C.G.: GW 6, (Collected Works 6) Walter-Verlag, Olten und Freiburg i.B..

Klöckner, J., Hartmann, T.: Der Wein erfreut des Menschen Herz. (Wine pleases the human heart) Paulus-Verlag, Freiburg 1999.

Kreuter, G.: Wein und Gesundheit, (Wine and Health) Heimat-Jahrbuch 59, Kreis Ahrweiler, 1997

Kroon, Ton van der .: Die Rückkehr des Löwen, von Liebe, Lust und Herzenspower, (The Return of the Lion, on love, lust and power of the heart) Verlag Hermann Bauer Freiburg, 3. Aufl., 2000.

Müller, K.-J.: Kopfkissen-Prüfung der Weinrebe Vitis vinifera. (Under-the-pillow proving of the Vine Vitis vinifera) Verlag Karl-Josef Müller, Zweibrücken 1997.

Opitz, W.: Sound of Wine. CD with sounds from different grape varieties during various stages of fermentation. Illmitz, 1996.

Pelikan, W.: Heilpflanzenkunde II (Healing Plants II). Philosophisch-anthropologischer Verlag, 2. Aufl., Goetheanum / Dornach, 1977.

Pryce, R. J., Langcake, P.: Alpha-Viniferin : An Antifungal Resveratrol Trimer from Grapevines. Phytochemistry 16 (1977) : 1452 – 1454.

Rätsch, C.: Enzyklopädie der psychoaktiven Pflanzen. (Encyclopaedia of Psychoactive Plants) AT Verlag, Aarau 1998.

Rätsch, C.: Heilkräuter der Antike, in Ägypten, Griechenland und Rom, (Healing Herbs in Classical Antiquity, in Egypt, Greeen and Rome) Eugen Diederichs Verlag, München 1995.

Rätsch, C.: Plants of Love, Ten Speed Press 1990.

Roberts, M.J.: Mythologie der Griechen und Römer, (Myths and Legends of Ancient Greece and Rome) Athenaion Verlag 1997.

Schlegel, E.: Religion der Arznei. (Religion of Medicine) Rohrmoser, Dresden 1915.

Scholten, J.: Homeopathy and the Elements. Stichting Alonnissos, Utrecht 1996.

Scholten, J.: Minerals in Plants, Stichting Alonnissos, Utrecht 2001.

Schroyens, F.: Synthesis: Repertorium Homoeopathicum Syntheticum, 7th edition, Homeopathic Book Publishers, London.

Sherr, J.: The Dynamics and Methodology of Homeopathic Provings. Dynamis Books, West Malvern 1994.

Stevens, A.: Das Phänomen C.G. Jung, (The Phenomenon of CG Jung) Biographische Wurzeln einer Lehre, Walther Verlag.

Steurer, R.: Gesundheit & Wein. (Health & Wine) Ueberreuter, Wien 2000.

Urania Enzyklopädie, Pflanzenreich, Blütenpflanzen 1 (Urania Encyclopaedia, Plant Kingdom, Flowering Plants 1).

Vithoulkas, G.: The Science of Homeopathy, Thorsons 1986.

Wunderer, W.:Rebschnitt für Könner. (Advanced Vine Pruning) In: Garten – Haus 9-10/2001. Österreichischer Agragverlag, Leopoldsdorf.

Edler Tropfen – Vom Werden des Weines: Ein Dokumentationsfilm von Interspot/ORF, 1998. (A Noble drop of Wine - On the Creation of Wine: A documentation film from Interspot/ORF, 1998)

Web sites:
http://www.wein-plus.de/weinfuehrer/index.html

Remedy suppliers:

Folium Vitis viniferae
Salvator-Apotheke in Eisenstadt (www.remedia.at) Robert Müntz.

Vitis vinifera cum fructibus
Löwen-Apotheke, Hauptstraße 93-95, 53340 Meckenheim, Tel. +49-2225-2256, Sven Göbel (C30-C200)
Salvator-Apotheke in Eisenstadt (www.remedia.at) Robert Müntz (C12, C30, C200, M, XM)

Other provings by the same authors

König, P., Swoboda, F.: Arzneimittelprüfung mit **Acidum succinicum** D30. In: Documenta Homoeopathica Bd 6. K.F.Haug Verlag, Heidelberg 1985.

König, P., Swoboda; F.: Erste Arzneimittelprüfung von **Magnesium fluoratum** D30. In: Documenta Homoeopathica Bd 8. K.F.Haug Verlag, Heidelberg 1987.

Swoboda, F., König, P.: Eine Arzneimittelprüfung mit **Ginkgo biloba** D30. In: Documenta Homoeopathica Bd 11. K.F.Haug Verlag, Heidelberg 1991.

König, P., Santos-König, U.: **Berberis**, **Rhododendron**, **Convallaria** – Traumgeschehen und Psychodynamik dreier Arzneiprüfungen. Burgdorf, Göttingen 1997.

Short biographies and authors' addresses

Peter König:

Born on 18.4.1955, in Laakirchen, Upper Austria. MD, University lecturer. Studied medicine in Graz and Vienna. First introduced to homeopathy through Mathias Dorcsi in 1978. Involved in lecturing, supervision, seminars and publication since 1983. On the committee of the Austrian Society for Homeopathic Medicine for 11 years. Lecturer at the 'Augsburger 3 month course' for Homeopathy since October 1993. Research associate at the 'Ludwig Boltzmann Institute for Homeopathy'. 1987-1990 Head of the homeopathic out-patient's department at the St Anna Children's Hospital in Vienna. 1990 - 2002 lectureship at the Faculty of Medicine at the University of Vienna (course of lectures on 'Introduction to Homeopathy'). Established own practice as GP from June 1987 in the 13th district in Vienna, later in Eichgraben, Lower Austria, and since 1999 in Eisenstadt. On the Editorial Board of the 'Homeopathic Links' journal since 1991. Publisher of 'Treating like with like - Homeopathy in Austria', Orac, 1996. 'Wisdoc' - Homeopathic EDP management system for documentation and patient details, in conjunction with Günther Nemeth, 1997-2001.

Now living in the wine producing area known as Burgenland I actually really love good (preferably heavy) red wines and up to now my connection with it has been more experiential rather than cognitive - and contrary to my true inclination I proved 'white' wine! - AUDE SAPERE!

Dr Peter König
Esterházyplatz 5
7000 Eisenstadt
0043-2682-72201
-72201-4 (Telefax)
koenigaudesapere@magnet.at
www.audesapere.com

Gerda Dauz:

Born on 23.03.1975 in St. Pölten, Austria. Studied medicine in Vienna, MD., practising in Linz, St. Pölten, Oberpullendorf and Eisenstadt. On maternity leave at present. Studying Classical Homeopathy since 1996.

Following numerous involuntary provings in the form of primary reaction after having been prescribed various high potency remedies, this Vitis vinifera proving is the first one for me that was intended as a proving - and in which I didn't develop any symptoms for a change. Could it be because I don't drink wine?

The assignement of looking for and finding identical and similar symptoms and themes in the various proving journals was certainly exciting, informative - and totally fitted in with my character ('conscientious about trifles'). I would like more of it!

Dr Gerda Dauz
Erlachgasse 126/52
1100 Wien
0044-664-1503664
Gerda.Dauz@gmx.at

Jürgen Weiland:

Co-incidence? Gerda Dauz and Peter König, who proved the leaf from the white grape, were both born in the spring. I was more drawn to the autumn and the black grape: I was born on 3rd October 1963 in Heimersheim/Ahr (in the romantic Ahrtal, not far from the German proving remedy's place of origin).

1981-1984 training to be a male nurse. From 1984 working as a male nurse, mainly in intensive care units and A & E as well as psychosomatic units. Trained to be a homeopath and alternative practitioner from 1989-1992, concluding my training at the Academy for Homeopathy in Gauting, near Munich. Own homeopathic practice in Bonn since 1992. College lecturer at the Centre for Classical Homeopathy, Mülheim/Ruhr, since 1993 and also visiting lecturer at the Academy for Homeopathy in Gautung (focusing on pregnancy - labour - post partum and infancy).

Involved in supervision and running study groups since 1996, in addition to homeopathy training for midwives. Managing a clinic at the 'Centre for Homeopathy and Obstetrics' in conjunction with the midwifery association Storch & Co. 1997-2000 further training in analytical psychology at the C.G. Jung Institute in Cologne.

Strong personal connection to the proving remedy from the Ahr region. It was a lengthy process, with a lot of time passing from the moment the idea was conceived to the final publication. My own personal process of development is tied in with it very much. The Spätburgunder had to mature for five whole years, before it could eventually be 'harvested' and made available.

Jürgen Weiland
Bonner Talweg 215
53129 Bonn
+49-228-263341
www.Juergen-Weiland.de
info@Juergen-Weiland.de

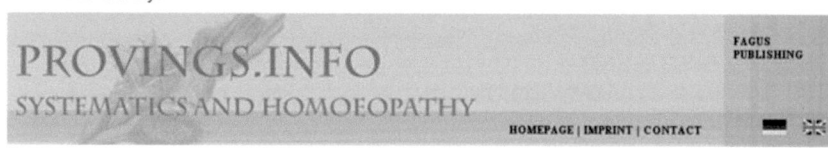